"The prickly pear is one of the most widespread cacti on Earth and has some of the most diverse uses, both as food and medicine. This book provides a comprehensive and detailed review of the benefits of this remarkable plant and a compelling argument for its increased acceptance into modern herbalism."

MARK BLUMENTHAL, EXECUTIVE DIRECTOR OF THE AMERICAN BOTANICAL COUNCIL AND EDITOR OF *HERBALGRAM*

"As an herbalist and ethnobotanist, I have scoured the literature to find more details about the use of these curious plants. My search has been rewarded by the publication of Ran Knishinsky's new book, *Prickly Pear Cactus Medicine*. He has done a masterful job unearthing details on the use of the prickly pear cactus for food and for medicine. This, the only cactus widely available in American supermarkets, is poised to become a dietary staple and Knishinsky's book provides the spark to move the prickly pear from beyond ethnic use to mainstream acceptance."

DAVID WINSTON, AHG, DEAN OF THE HERBAL THERAPEUTICS SCHOOL OF BOTANICAL MEDICINE AND CHAIR OF THE ADMISSIONS REVIEW COMMITTEE FOR THE AMERICAN HERBALIST GUILD

"A wonderful book about a wonderful herb. An excellent blend of good science and real life applications showing the relevance of prickly pear in the treatment of conditions such as diabetes, cholesterol management and a range of immunological problems. The wealth of gourmet recipes and practical guidelines will prove invaluable to the many people that prickly pear will benefit."

DAVID HOFFMANN, FNIMH, AHG,
R OF *MEDICAL HERBALISM* AND
LLUSTRATED *HOLISTIC HERBAL*

D1010012

Also by Ran Knishinsky

The Clay Cure
Natural Healing From the Earth

The Prozac Alternative
Natural Relief from Depression with
St. John's Wort, Kava, Ginkgo, 5-HTP, Homeopathy,
and Other Alternative Therapies

Prickly Pear

Cactus Medicine

Treatments for Diabetes,
Cholesterol,
and the Immune System

Ran Knishinsky

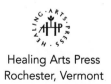

Healing Arts Press
Rochester, Vermont

Healing Arts Press
One Park Street
Rochester, Vermont 05767
www.InnerTraditions.com

Healing Arts Press is a division of Inner Traditions International

Copyright © 2004 by Ran Knishinsky

All rights reserved. No part of this book may be reproduced or utilized
in any form or by any means, electronic or mechanical, including pho-
tocopying, recording, or by any information storage and retrieval system, without permission in writing from the publisher.

*Note to the reader: This book is intended as an informational guide.
The remedies, approaches, and techniques described herein are meant
to supplement, and not to be a substitute for, professional medical care
or treatment. They should not be used to treat a serious ailment without prior consultation with a qualified health care professional.*

Library of Congress Cataloging-in-Publication Data
Knishinsky, Ran, 1971–
  Prickly pear cactus medicine : treatments for diabetes, cholesterol,
and the immune system / Ran Knishinsky.
    p. cm.
  Includes bibliographical references and index.
  ISBN 978-0-89281-149-6 (pbk.)
  1. Prickly pears—Therapeutic use. I. Title.
  RS165.P73K658 2004
  615'.32356—dc22

                                                        2004003633

Printed and bound in the United States

10 9 8 7 6 5 4 3 2

Text design by Virginia Scott-Bowman
Text layout by Mary Anne Hurhula
This book was typeset in Sabon

Contents

Preface vii

1 Cactus Medicine 1

2 What Is a Cactus? 14

3 The Healing Parts of the
Prickly Pear Cactus 20

4 The Cactus-Diabetes Connection 29

5 The Cactus-Cholesterol Connection 55

6 Other Benefits of and Treatments
Using Prickly Pear Cactus 67

7 Application and Dosage of
Prickly Pear Cactus 80

8 Picking and Preparing the Prickly Pear 87

9 Cactus Cooking 98

APPENDIX A Prickly Pear Suppliers 112

APPENDIX B Herbal Education and
Natural Product Services 119

APPENDIX C General Resources for Diabetes and
Heart Disease 122

Notes 126

Bibliography 135

Preface

Prickly Pear Cactus Medicine is the first complete guide to the natural medicinal benefits of the prickly pear cactus. It summarizes the literature and research on an herb that is now considered a wonder medicine by researchers and herbalists. It provides an up-close and in-depth examination of how this medicine is utilized from the perspective of the doctor, chemist, ethnobotanist, cook, and layperson. It also provides an introduction to the desert, home of the prickly pear. Cactus recipes are included in the text for the discriminating and adventurous palate. There is also an extensive reference and notes section that will guide you to resources that were utilized in preparing this book.

To learn more about the health benefits of cactus eating and to locate different sources of fruits, flowers, and pads in your area please visit my Web site:

www.cactusmedicine.com

Cactus Medicine

*The use of traditional remedies was highly pragmatic and
the Seri (Native American people) generally did not have
specific explanations for the efficacy of their medicines.
When asked why a particular remedy was used, the usual
answer was "because it works."*
—Richard Stephen Felger and Mary Beck Moser,
*People of the Desert and Sea:
Ethnobotany of the Seri Indians*[1]

The prickly pear cactus has enjoyed an element of popularity
unlike any other plant in the herbal kingdom. Its unique
shape, form, and usage have earned it a title of distinction
among other herbs. Its long history of use is reflected in Native
American, and particularly Aztec, legends in which the prickly
pear is a central figure. The cactus forms part of the Mexican
national shield that appears on the country's flag, and in Texas
the fruit has been dubbed the official state plant. Proving its
enduring popularity the prickly pear has recently made
appearances in Snapple Iced Teas in the form of a prickly
pear–flavored bottled tea and in a prickly pear–flavored mar-
garita at the Chevy's Mexican restaurant chain.

The prickly pear cactus is unique among other plants,
and even among other cacti. Very few plants in the botanical
kingdom are a vegetable, fruit, and flower all in one. The

Spanish conquerors of Mexico recognized the benefits of the prickly pear fruits, due to their vitamin C content, as a partial cure for the scurvy that plagued their sailors.[2] The Aztec leader Montezuma II might have been enjoying a nice hot cup of chocolate when the Spanish arrived, but there was probably a plate of prickly pear pads sitting in one of his many kitchens, waiting to be served.[3] The prickly pear has persisted as a staple food in the diets of those native to the southwestern portion of the United States and those settled throughout Central and South America and even in parts of Europe and the Middle East.

The driving force behind the prickly pear's use and popularity is its ability to function as both food and medicine. Because of the cactus's striking ability to thrive in some of the most harsh desert habitats, it has represented to desert inhabitants, especially those in the southwestern United States and Central America, an alternative to death in an often brutal environment. But the prickly pear was not only valued as a reliable source of food and drink; it was also treasured for its health benefits. At a time when antibiotics like penicillin and vaccinations did not exist, the cactus was an herbal prescription for the sick and healthy alike. Current scientific research is validating what ancestral cultures learned about the prickly pear: it is a healer.

BOTANICAL POSSIBILITIES

The use of unadulterated, nontoxic medicines is gaining favor among scientists, physicians, and lay users. In 1990, the *New England Journal of Medicine* reported that more than one-third of all Americans had visited an alternative practitioner at one time. More than a decade later, it is fascinating to recognize the ever growing presence of natural therapies for the treatment of acute and chronic disorders. Despite the commer-

TABLE 1.1. CURRENT FOCUS OF PRICKLY PEAR MEDICAL RESEARCH

Management and treatment of type II diabetes

Useful in the treatment of hyperlipidemias

Anti-inflammatory action

Useful in the management of obesity

Investigation of antiviral properties

Potential cancer prevention agent for specific cancers

Wound-healing properties

Treats symptoms of BPH

cial popularity of pharmaceuticals, natural remedies are finding their place at the bedside once again.

For centuries, the mechanism of action behind the healthful effects of botanical medicine has been hotly debated among both scientists and traditional herbalists. In response to the public's increasing demand for natural remedies, esteemed medical institutions have turned their attention to alternative medical practices such as botanical medicine. An increasing number of published studies have helped to validate the therapeutic agents and the beneficial physiological effects of plants. Pharmaceutical companies, both phyto-pharmaceuticals and traditional-pharmaceuticals, have played active roles in researching, developing, and promoting herbal medications. Interestingly, this resurgence in herbal use is attributable in large part to the increased amount of scientific investigation of herbs that is currently being undertaken by the medical establishment, and not as a direct result of the traditional herbalists movement.

THE TRADITIONAL HERBALIST VERSUS MODERN SCIENCE

Prior to our current, more scientific understanding of the mechanism of action behind herbs, traditional herbalists postulated their own empyreal explanations. Throughout the Middle Ages, illness was often attributed to the presence of evil spirits. Herbs were supposedly endowed with magical and spiritual powers that were capable of ridding individuals of these evil spirits and nursing them back to health. By today's definition, this theory seems somewhat archaic. But for centuries, traditional herbalists maintained that a botanical herb consists of latent spiritual energy that acts as the one primary healing property. This energy force was believed by some to contain the essence of a higher spirit. The herb imparted its energy force to the person or animal that consumed it. Healing then occurred on two levels: the spiritual and the physical.

In addition, it was thought that the life force that existed within the herb was largely characteristic of the plant's physical habitat. The herb imparted a healing power that was reminiscent of its particular character and its relationship to nature. For instance, the prickly pear cactus, endowed with adaptive qualities that allow it to thrive in the most difficult climatic and environmental conditions, was thought to increase the body's level of resistance to disease. Furthermore, believers in the Doctrine of Signatures, an ancient theory that every plant bears a clear sign of its use, might interpret the thorns of the prickly pear cactus as symbolic of its defensive posture, indicating the plant's usefulness as a healer of wounds.

Given the radical developments in medicine over the last century, most modern herbalists have discarded these ethereal theories in favor of a more scientific understanding. Others have integrated traditional theories with a twenty-first century approach to medicine, developing a quasi-spiritualized scientific theory of the mechanism of action behind botanical medicine.

Certainly, the scientific establishment offers a far more structured and evidence-based theory to explain an herb's success in healing. Today's researcher is equipped with sophisticated technology making it possible to discover the medicinal agents within a plant. Plants, each unique in their size, shape, and chemical makeup, are made up of compounds commonly referred to as *phytonutrients* (*phyto* is the Greek word for plant). In scientific literature, phytonutrients have been reported to act as enzymes, pigments, and growth regulators in plants as well as providing odor, color, and taste. They are also involved in protecting the plant from potentially harmful and deadly bacteria, viruses, injuries, and insects. Since these active chemicals are responsible for the maintenance of the plant's life, it is not surprising that they demonstrate therapeutic activity in the laboratory and in controlled studies with humans. These compounds help regulate vital body processes to maintain health and assist in the fight against disease.

PHYTOCHEMICALS AND FLAVONOIDS

Phytochemicals

The discovery of phytonutrients, also referred to as phytochemicals, in plants has been hailed as one of the most significant findings in herbal research. The study of these compounds and their application in medicine has shaped our understanding of how herbs operate in the human body. Single crude herbs are made of numerous phytochemicals. Each chemical is partly or wholly responsible for a specific function. However, the chemical diversity and variability of components within the crude herb is somewhat baffling to the medical establishment because the chemical structure of herbs directly contrasts that of modern laboratory-generated drugs.[4] Unlike their herbal counterparts, pharmaceutical drugs, when naturally derived, are usually single molecular entities consisting of one isolated, purified chemical.[5]

The existence of multiple agents within a given herb is thought to offer many advantages. First, because of the broad range of constituents with an herb, herbs are typically employed in a multifunctional manner in the treatment of one or more ailments. Second, it is thought by some herbalists that the emergence of new disease and patient targets expands the role of some agents within the herb. Those agents that might have been previously identified as inactive may later assume a role of greater proportion. Third, it is hypothesized that multiple constituents within the herb have crossover functions capable of treating disease and its evolutionary mutations. This latter point is controversial and is the subject of ongoing debate. Nevertheless, the medical establishment acknowledges the complex presence of varying, sometimes seemingly unrelated, compounds as a unique characteristic of botanical medicine.

Table 1.2 lists various phytochemicals in selected common herbs and the specific immunological action the herb performs. There are often multiple constituents responsible for the medicine's total therapeutic benefit; however, for the purposes of this book, only one is listed for each.

Flavonoids

There are many different compounds in the prickly pear cactus, several of which are highlighted in this book. Currently the best recognized compounds in the cactus are the flavonoids. Abundant in the cactus, *flavonoids* are a group of biologically active molecules that fall under the umbrella classification of phytochemicals. Under this umbrella, the class belongs to the polyphenol family.[6] Polyphenols are found in high concentrations in wine, tea, grapes, and a wide variety of other plants. To date, at least 8,000 phenolic compounds have been identified in a dozen chemical subcategories.[7] Included in the polyphenol

TABLE 1.2
HERBAL PHYTOCHEMICALS

HERB	PHYTOCHEMICAL	THERAPEUTIC EFFECT
St. John's Wort	Xanthone	Partly responsible for antidepressant, antimicrobial, antiviral, and diuretic actions
Echinacea	Polysaccharides	Immunostimulatory & mild antiinflammatory effect
Ginger	Gingerol	Shows potent cardiotonic activity
Grapeseed Extract	Procyanidolic olignmer extract	Treatment of venous & capillary disorders including venous insufficiency and capillary fragility
Mistletoe	Lectin I	Potent inducer of cytokines such as interleukin 1, interleukin 6, and tumor necrosis factor
Onion	Allyl popyl disulfide	Active blood sugar-lowering agent
Peppermint	Menthol	External analgesic
Siberian Ginseng	Eleutherosides	Responsible for the adaptogenic effect
Valerian	Valepotriates	Partly responsible for sedative effects

Source: Michael T. Murray, N.D., The Healing Power of Herbs, and Roy Upton, et al. American Herbal Pharmacopoeia and Therapeutic Compendium. "St. John's wort: Hypericum perforatum," Santa Cruz, 1997, 9.

classification are the flavonoids, of which the best known are the bioflavonoids (other better known biologically active flavonoid compounds include *catcehin, epicatechin, epicatechin gallate, epigallocatechin gallate,* and *proanthocyanidins*).[8]

Flavonoids impart the colorful pigment to fruits, vegetables, and herbs. They are responsible for the red, yellow, and orange colors of many flowers including prickly pear flowers, and also of many fruits including cactus fruits. Flavonoids can also be found in legumes, grains, and nuts. The rinds of citrus fruits are a rich source of flavonoid compounds, including *rutin* and *hespirdin,* and are perhaps the most familiar.

Widespread research on the biological action of flavonoids has recently burgeoned. The following is a sampling of some of the recently discovered applications of flavonoids:

- Age-related vision disorders: Given flavonoids' free-radical scavenging activity and their inhibitory effects on select free radicals, they are capable of helping to prevent damage to connective tissue framework surrounding capillary walls.[9] Thus, flavonoids have been credited with preventing macular degeneration and fighting cataracts presumably via an ability to deliver blood and oxygen to the eye.[10]

- Antiviral, anti-inflammatory, and antihistamine: Flavonoid consumption prevents the release and synthesis of compounds that promote inflammation in the joints and muscles as a result of fibromyalgia, gout, arthritis, exercise, and allergies.[11,12]

- Cancer: Flavonoid compounds in such herbs as green tea, soy, grapeseed extract, and pycnogenol have been credited with lowering the risk of certain types of cancer (breast, prostate, stomach, pancreatic, lung) due to their ability to exert antioxidant actions by inhibiting the activities of pro-oxidant enzymes.

- Cardiovascular: Biologically active flavonoids help to normalize blood platelet stickiness, allowing the blood to flow more smoothly through the important vessels, and thereby are an important nutritional factor in maintaining proper cardiovascular health and managing microvascular disorders.[13] According to recent studies, tea drinking may help heart-attack victims survive. That's because flavonoids also have many potential clinical applications including the restoration of normal blood vessel function, according to a recent article published in the May 2002 issue of the medical journal *Circulation*.[14] Researchers at Beth Israel Deaconess Medical Center in Boston followed 1,900 heart-attack patients for nearly four years and found those who drank two or more cups of tea per day reduced their risk of death by 44 percent, compared with non-tea drinkers.[15]

- Diabetes mellitus: In Europe, flavonoids have been used in the prevention and treatment of diabetic retinopathy.[16] Also, their ability to reduce plasma LDL cholesterol coupled with a protective effect on capillary fragility has been put to use in the treatment of this disorder.

- Antioxidant: The oxidant reactions of free radicals, molecules with unpaired electrons, have been linked to many chronic and degenerative diseases including heart disease, arthritis, and cancer, in addition to the aging process. The human body is constantly subject to attacks by free radicals, which can destroy cell membrane lipids and damage DNA.[17] Attacked from both within and without, the body creates its own antioxidant compounds, such as the enzyme *superoxide dismutase* (SOD), to combat the free radicals. However, the body is incapable of producing other types of antioxidants such as vitamins C, E, beta-carotene, and certain flavonoids, many of which are obtained through multiple servings of fruits and vegetables.

Experimental studies with flavonoids have demonstrated their ability to reverse the oxidation process and help prevent free-radical formation.[18] Flavonoids achieve this through a multiple number of mechanisms of action. At present, scientists have identified at least six different possible antioxidant mechanisms of flavonoids.[19]

1. Direct radical scavenging: Flavonoids may act at any stage of the radical developmental process. For instance, they might trap hydroxyl free radicals.
2. Down-regulation of radical production: The flavonoids react with peroxy radicals to slow their propagation and delay the onset of lipid peroxidation.[20]
3. Elimination of radical precursors: Flavonoids proactively work to eliminate the precursors to free radicals, such as hydrogen peroxide, thus eliminating them before a problem ensues.
4. Metal chelation: Flavonoids prevent radical formation by chelation of transition metals such as iron, preventing iron-induced lipid peroxidation.[21]
5. Inhibition of xanthine oxidase: Flavonoids act as antioxidants by inhibiting *prooxidant enzymes,* such as xanthine oxidase, the most prominent example, which can, in certain states, contribute to the production of superoxide radicals.[22]
6. Elevation of endogenous antioxidants: Flavonoids elevate body concentrations of endogenous antioxidants (antioxidants that are produced within the body), such as SOD (superoxide dismutase), which themselves eliminate free radicals or their precursors. The flavonoids also serve to inhibit the damaging effects of enzymes that can degrade connective tissue structures or prevent their depletion.[23]

Taking Phytochemicals

Most of the studies on the benefits of phytochemical consumption involve intake of phytochemical-rich foods or herbs, not isolated phytochemical extracts. For instance, most sources of flavonoids will elicit the same basic biochemical response, but in varying degrees according to the naturally present levels of the various flavonoid compound(s) in the food. The quantity and quality of the respective phytonutrient content is dependent not only upon the source, but also upon the variety of species, quality of soil, maturity, and method of preparation. Not all phytochemical compounds are created equal. Products on the marketplace will vary according to their level of phytonutrient content and quality.

Standardized extracts are one way of assuring the quality of an herb in terms of its active components. A standardized extract, commonly referred to as a guaranteed potency extract, is an extract guaranteed to contain a standardized level of active principles.[24] When the content of active compounds is certified it provides the greatest degree of consistency and assurance of quality per capsule or serving, depending on the delivery system. An extract alone does not mean that it has been isolated from the other so-called inactive factors, however. A standardized extract of the prickly pear flowers for its polyphenol content, say at 12 percent, still contains all those synergistic factors that enhance the function of the active ingredient. This is one benefit to purchasing a standardized extract of an herb. Oral intake of a crude herb or standardized extract in a bed of the crude herb might therefore be preferred to the consumption of an isolated extract.

Research has shown that the combination of whole-food ingredients may be more effective than just a single phytochemical. As an example, vitamin C plus flavonoids might be more effective than either compound alone.[25] This is why some naturopaths would suggest drinking the flower tea rather than consuming a pure, isolated flavonoid extract from the flower petals. The absorption and metabolism of the flavonoids may depend on other food components naturally present. The alcohol in red wine, by way of illustration, may make flavonoids more biologically active than they would be without the alcohol. The same concept holds true for the prickly pear cactus fruits. Consumption of the nectar or jelly prepared from the whole fruit, for example, is preferable to an isolated extract of flavonoid or pectin from the fruit given other compounds present that might exert a synergistic effect.

Herbal Prescription Drugs

The history of clinical pharmacology is characterized by the incremental improvements in the safety, efficacy, selectivity, and utility of a single chemical. Some critics look at the incremental advances as being too costly, and criticize them as having no significant differences from the original agent. However, pharmaceutical companies argue that the new medicines that emerge from this evolutionary process can offer advantages in terms of cost savings, more patient satisfaction, compliance, and improved efficacy.[26]

Despite the stark contrast between multiconstituent herbs and their single-component synthetic counterparts, herbal active ingredients have found their way into the pharmacopoeia of Food and Drug Administration (FDA)–approved prescription drugs. Herbal phytonutrients have been standardized and in some cases synthesized.[27] You might be surprised to find that one-fourth of all prescription drugs sold in the United States contain active constituents obtained from plants. In fact, the World Health Organization notes that of 119 plant-derived pharmaceutical medicines, about 74 percent are used by modern medicines in ways that correlate directly with their traditional use as plant medicines by native cultures.[28] Further, an estimated $11 billion worth of plant-based medicines are sold in the United States every year and $43 billion worldwide.[29]

Examples of isolated, purified compounds once derived from herbs are numerous and include:

- Colchicine, used to treat attacks of gout, is a drug originally derived from *Colchicum autumnale,* autumn crocus.[30]
- Digoxin, used to treat congestive heart failure, is a drug originally derived from the foxglove plant, *Digitalis lanata.*[31]
- Morphine, a drug whose primary clinical use is in the management of moderately severe and severe pain, was originally derived from the opium poppy, *Papaver somniafera.*[32]
- Reserpine, prescribed for mild to moderate hypertension, was originally developed from Indian snakeroot, *Rauvolfia serpentina.*[33]

Even some OTC (over-the-counter) medicines, such as those for sleep, cold, headache, weight loss, constipation, and nausea, feature active herbal chemical constituents. Most people don't realize this when they purchase these products at the drugstore because the herbs are usually listed in their complicated Latin nomenclatures and are easily overlooked. The presence of herbs plays a greater role in our lives than most of us realize.

What Is a Cactus?

The enigma of the desert is its life.
—William G. McGinnies, Ph.D.

THE CACTUS FAMILY

The cactus family is one of approximately 350 families of flowering plants. Cacti belong to one of the youngest plant families, and probably because of their rose-shaped flowers are thought to descend from the rose family.[1] Though it is often hard to see this similarity through the thorns and rough texture of a cactus, the plant in full bloom reveals some of these traits.

The cactus family is divided into three subfamilies based on growth form, which are further divided into species. The family contains roughly two thousand species in ninety-five genera, or main groups. The number of species and their names change as scientists learn more about cacti.

Cacti are referred to in the scientific literature as succulents. You may be familiar with the term *succulent* since one of the most famous herbs in the natural products industry, aloe vera, belongs to this group. A succulent is a desert plant, with extensive adaptations against water loss. In other words, cacti store water like a sponge to protect their water supply. Since all cactus habitats experience periodic droughts, the plants draw on this reserve when water is scarce.

A cactus takes in water through a widespread, shallow root system that is ready to absorb water whenever it comes, even from mist or a light rain. In a harsh desert habitat, it's imperative that the plant can rapidly replenish its water supply quickly and efficiently.[2] Once absorbed, the moisture is drawn up into the storage cells of the plant, where the cactus chemically changes it into a mucilaginous substance, which does not evaporate as fast as the thin, watery sap usually found in large-leafed plants.[3]

The cactus stem has a thick, waxy covering that helps seal in moisture, thus preventing water loss by evaporation. As a result, prickly pear joints swell up when they are holding an abundance of water. The joints then contract during periods of drought when the cactus must live off its storage. Thus, the cactus can be a precious source of liquid in a desert emergency.

EVERY CACTUS HAS ITS THORNS

Most cacti have thorns—if you do not already know this, once you touch a few cacti, you will learn very quickly. Sometimes only lightly brushing up against a cactus can be enough to dislodge a thorn. Other times it takes quite a bit of pushing and pulling. If you are ever the unlucky recipient of a cactus thorn in your side, expect a little pain, but do not worry about any permanent damage. There is no such thing as a poisonous thorn. In fact, if a thorn ever sticks you, the chances are very good that the pad from which the thorn came could heal your wound!

Cacti spines are modified leaves that serve several adaptive functions. Spines can be hard, soft, curved, hooked, round, stiff, papery, hairlike, or even feathery. They are mostly recognized as a deterrent to thirsty, browsing animals. But cacti do not use their thorns exclusively as weapons. Sometimes they can be a means of transportation to another locale. If a cactus thorn lodges on you, it could be the thorn's way of saying, "Hey, stranger, give me a ride." When you dislodge the cactus joint at another location, it will take root and spring into a new plant.[4]

The cacti spines also provide substantial shade and serve as points to radiate heat. This keeps their body as much as 10 degrees cooler than it would otherwise be. A difference of 10 degrees is enormous in the desert. The spines also help to break up wind, reducing its drying effect on the pads. Cacti prefer to grow thorns instead of leaves because leaves draw additional water from the plant without any of the other previously mentioned benefits. It is an example of the evolution of plants.

OPUNTIA BY ANY OTHER NAME

Opuntia streptacantha, Neomammillaria micocarpa, Coryphantha vivipara, Ferocactus viridescens. In case you are wondering, these are the Latin names that botanists use for various kinds of cacti. The scientific name of a plant is constructed like the name of a person, but with the surname first. The surname of the prickly pear cactus, for example, is *Opuntia*. The surname for the giant cactus is *Cereus,* and the surname for the hedgehog cactus is *Echinocereus*.

The cactus genus we are concerned with is the group *Opuntia* (pronounced O-pun-TEE-yuh). This group has the greatest number of species and the most variation in form, size, coloration, and habit of growth than any other group. They require no cultivation or irrigation and can withstand some of the harshest climatic changes. The two major branches of the *Opuntia* genus are the prickly pears and the chollas (pronounced CHOY-yahs). The prickly pears are known for their flattened stems (sometimes referred to as joints or pads) that grow out of one another.

Plants are not classified by their individual traits, but rather by what each plant in a family has in common with the other in that family. One common characteristic of the opuntia group is that each species has small "bunches" of hair, or bristles, that grow along the top of each wart. These are called *glochids* (pronounced GLOW-kids).[5] While an opuntia may not have thorns, it could be covered by glochids. They are so tiny, sometimes as fine as peach fuzz, that they can be difficult to remove and very prickly to the touch, often making them more troublesome than the spines.

A major difference between the two opuntia families is the manner in which they hold their joints. Prickly pears develop a network of fibers to hold their pads in shape. That is why their stems can be cut through with ease. Chollas, on the other hand, develop a woody stem within their joints for strength, making them nearly impossible to cut apart.

Another difference is the edibility of the fruits, that grow from the two families. The fruit of the prickly pear is a pleasant-tasting treat, much like watermelon except with pulp and small, hard black seeds. The fruit that belongs to the cholla, on the other hand, is not quite as tasty. In fact, it is downright horrible.

Yet another difference between the two families of cacti is what is inside the pads and joints. The prickly pear contains a bitter and somewhat sticky juice that can be pressed or sucked from the insides of the stems. As I mentioned before, this liquid substance can be used as emergency water or as an active healing agent. However, the joints of the cholla cannot be utilized for the same healing purposes as the prickly pear because of their woody stem and their lack of mucilaginous material.

THE HOME OF THE PRICKLY PEAR

Thanks to its durability and adaptability the prickly pear has achieved wider distribution than any other group of plants in the cactus family. They can be found on bare or grassy plains, on high cold mountains, in jungles, along seashores, in subtropical areas, as well as in arid and semiarid regions.

Perhaps its most famous and well-recognized home is the desert. After all, when we think of the desert we think of cacti.

And when we think of cacti we think of the desert. But how the desert supports life, both animal and plant, is shrouded in mystery. Most people have a very rudimentary understanding of the desert. People who visit the desert for the first time expect to see a barren wasteland, similar to the Sahara: a lifeless, rainless, sandy, and inhospitable piece of land. However, most deserts in the world are more like a botanical garden.

The Sonoran desert, located in the southwest portion of the United States, one of the most well-known and popular homes to the cactus, is a vibrant display of life. Spread over thousands of square miles of valleys and plateaus, the vast desert floor is covered with an even layer of egg-sized rocks. Jagged mountains create the backdrop for a vast display of desert botany, which include different types of cacti, trees, and shrubs. Each varies in color to such a degree that it is common to see twenty to thirty shades of colors in any one-mile span of unadulterated desert. There are places in the desert where the botanical life imitates jungle life. Plants sit on each other's laps, growing in-between one another, in a lavish display of strangely contorted foliage that captures the imagination. Some of these plants look as if they have persisted since long before the prehistoric age.[6]

Still, scientists are not really sure how or why life exists in the desert. Our notion of the desert's living things, their form, and how they function was formulated from experiences and observations in tropical and temperate climates.[7] When scientists first stumbled upon the desert habitat, complete with desert plant and animal life, they were surprised and confused. Desert plants, especially cactus plants like the prickly pear, function like any other plant in the botanical kingdom. They manufacture their own food, and control their own growth and reproduction.[8] They also possess the ability to adapt to the environment in which they live.

Ironically, while prickly pears grow in more places in the world than any other cacti, they are the most short-lived of all cacti. Seldom does an individual prickly pear live more than twenty years. Despite their short life span, these cacti propagate quickly, easily regenerating from pads, root calluses, and seeds.

The prickly pear cactus is a living representative of a race of plants that has undergone the greatest evolution in entering the desert and have acquired all the characteristics that have made possible their survival and success. Prickly pears are considered by some botanists to be the hardiest, most adaptable plants in the cactus family.[9] Furthermore, the prickly pear is a perennial plant, which means that it grows all year long. Cultivated all over the world in such areas as Africa (including as far north as Morocco and as far south as South Africa), Italy, Israel, Spain, the United States, Mexico, Colombia, Brazil, Peru, Bolivia, Chile, and Argentina, the cactus is readily available. As such, it has become increasingly researched as a food source and as a medicine.

The Healing Parts of the Prickly Pear Cactus

An old woman atop the hill throwing out old tortillas . . .
—Mexican riddle describing the
shape of the prickly pear

The prickly pear cactus is unique among cacti, and in fact among all plants, in that each part of the plant may be used for some healthful purpose. Though you may never have come face to face with a prickly pear, chances are you have probably seen one before. They range in height from as small as 6 inches to as large as 12 feet tall. The pad, commonly referred to as nopal, (or *nopales* in Spanish), is the source of many vitamins, minerals, and amino acids. The fruit of the cactus—also known as tuna in the Spanish vernacular, and nicknamed by others Indian fig and cactus pear—contains adequate amounts of pectin and vitamins. The flowers, which grow from the fruit, are well recognized for their flavonoid properties. Each part of the prickly pear anatomy and their basic uses are detailed in the following sections.

CACTUS PADS

Green, spiny, thickened stems form the body of the prickly pear plant. The joints, or pads, range in size and shape—some have "beaver tail"-shaped joints as small as the human ear, while others have joints as large as a four hundred-page textbook. Sometimes these pads, regardless of the shape, grow toward the sky. Other pads lie on the dirt, forming a desert carpet. The uniform color of the prickly pear pads is green, but the shades vary from faint light green to light purple.

Vitamin and Mineral Content

The modest cactus pads of the prickly pear are a storehouse of nutrients. They include a healthy dose of the minerals potassium, magnesium, calcium, and iron.[1] They are also particularly high in the dietary antioxidant vitamin A (in the form of beta-carotene), in levels comparable to spinach, and high in antioxidant vitamin C. Antioxidants are agents that restrict the deleterious effects of oxidant reactions within the body. Daily intake of antioxidants has shown to be effective in preventing the oxidation of arterial cholesterol and reversing arterial damage. In chapter 5, I will explore the role of antioxidants on plasma LDL cholesterol concentrations.

Amino Acids

The pads also contain a full range of amino acids, the building blocks of protein, including the eight essential amino acids not manufactured by the body. The benefits of amino acid consumption are far-reaching, as protein is involved in multiple chemical interactions within the body. It is extremely rare that a plant source provides such a high and broad composition of amino acids as the prickly pear. Its utility as a nutritional, high-fiber, low-fat food is amplified by this unique and exquisite amino acid profile. Vegans and vegetarians who rely on legumes such as soybeans and peas to fulfill their protein requirements will find in the nopal pads a source of high-quality protein.[2]

TABLE 3.1. NUTRITIONAL PROFILE
OF THE PRICKLY PEAR PADS

Quantities given are based on amount per 100 grams of prickly pear.
(100 grams = approx 1.25 cups)

Calories	16
Fat (grams)	trace
Cholesterol (milligrams)	0
Carbohydrates (grams)	3.3
Dietary fiber (grams)	2.3
Protein (grams)	1.2
MINERALS	
Calcium (milligrams)	163
Iron (milligrams)	0.7
Magnesium (milligrams)	58
Phosphorus (milligrams)	17
Potassium (milligrams)	319
Sodium (milligrams)	22
Copper (milligrams)	0.06
Selenium (micrograms)	0.7
Zinc (milligrams)	0.3
VITAMINS	
Vitamin C (milligrams)	13
Thiamin (milligrams)	0.01
Riboflavin (milligrams)	0.04
Niacin (milligrams)	0.5
Vitamin B_6 (milligrams)	0.07
Folate (micrograms)	3
Vitamin B_{12} (micrograms)	0
Vitamin A (I.U.)	415
Vitamin E (A.T.E.)	0.002

Source: U.S. Department of Agriculture Nutrient Database

TABLE 3.2. AMINO ACID PROFILES
(mg/g of dehydrated nopal)

ESSENTIAL AMINO ACIDS	
Histidine	0.08
Isoleucine	2.53
Leucine	5.14
Lysine	4.50
Methionine	0.80
Phenylalanine	2.88
Threonine	1.38
Valine	4.31
NON-ESSENTIAL AMINO ACIDS	
Alanine	3.95
Arginine	1.26
Aspartic acid	0.32
Cysteine	0.16
Glutamic acid	1.66
Glycine	4.50
Proline	3.48
Serine	0.36
Tyrosine	2.05

Source: Assad Kazeminy Ph.D., Laboratory Director, "Sample Description: Dehydrated Nopal." Streptacantha sample: 7/07/1994 provided by Cactulife.

Medicinal Benefits

Many people from Mexico and Central and South America have traditionally used medicinal plants to control a variety of illnesses, including hyperglycemia.[3] This trend continues today. In the March/April 2002 issue of the *Journal of the American Pharmaceutical Association*, a study on the use of herbal products for diabetes by Latinos was published. The authors of the study recognized the prickly pear cactus as one of the most extensively studied herbal hypoglycemics in addition to its use as a common food in the Latin American diet. Patients were asked whether they used nopal as a hypoglycemic agent, as a food source only, or both; most reported using nopal for both purposes, and only a low percentage used it as a food source only. On average these patients reported consuming nopal once every other day. They eat nopal as part of their regular diet or when they feel their glucose levels are high.[4]

Recent medical studies on the prickly pear cactus pads have explored and verified their use as an "antidiabetic" remedy. Studies published in the *Journal of Ethnopharmacology* and *Diabetes Care* have documented the effectiveness of prickly pear pads' use in the treatment of individuals with type II diabetes. Results of the studies have yielded strong positive results showing a noticeable hypoglycemic effect in patients with non-insulin-dependent diabetes mellitus (NIDDM).[5] A decrease in glucose absorption and an improvement in insulin response were also noted in these studies. Further research has successfully demonstrated that the high content of flavonoids in pads contributes to their ability to reduce undesirable low-density lipids—otherwise known as the "bad" cholesterol. Chapter 4, "The Cactus-Diabetes Connection," explores the antidiabetic clinical studies and investigates the use of different species of prickly pear cactus to treat and manage diabetes.

According to Charles W. Weber, professor of nutritional sciences at the University of Arizona, perhaps the most important component in the cactus is its dietary soluble fiber, which comes especially in the mucilage and pectin.[6] Mucilage is the sticky juice that oozes from the pad when it is sliced. In medical circles, this sticky substance is referred to as *mucilaginous polysaccharide*. Interestingly, polysaccharides are the primary active ingredient of other popular immune-stimulating herbs such as aloe vera, echinacea, astragalus, and Asian mushrooms.

CACTUS FRUITS

At the end of summer the joints produce their tiny fruit. The color and size of the fruit differs according to the species. The color of the fruit can range from green to red to purple. Their size is somewhat consistent, measuring from 2 to 4 inches in length and 1 to 2 inches in diameter. It is similar in shape to the kiwi, and comes in its own convenient wrapper.

The fruit is one of the tastiest parts of the prickly pear. Although low in calories, it is apt to satisfy the sweetest tooth and therefore makes an ideal treat for those watching their waistline. It can be picked off the cactus and eaten raw or prepared in many different ways (see chapter 9 for cactus recipes).

Prickly pear fruit is becoming increasingly available in the United States in grocery and specialty stores. It is farmed and exported from several countries including Mexico, Colombia, Chile, Honduras, Israel, Nicaragua, and Italy. When available, it is generally offered for sale both fresh and dried.

In Israel, where exportation of the cactus fruits has grown into a large, commercially successful business, the fruit is referred to as a *sabrah*. Interestingly, the word *sabrah* is also used to identify a person born in the land of Israel. According to local folklore, like the prickly pear fruit, the people of Israel have a rough exterior but are tremendously sweet and soft inside.

Vitamin and Mineral Content

The fruit is packed with cofactors that boost immunity. It contains significant portions of the minerals calcium, magnesium, and potassium. It also contains a large proportion of antioxidant compounds, including flavonoids. Antioxidants are agents that restrict the deleterious effects of oxidant reactions within the body. Daily intake of antioxidants has shown to be effective in preventing the oxidation of arterial cholesterol and reversing arterial damage, in addition to helping protect

TABLE 3.3. NUTRITIONAL PROFILE
OF THE PRICKLY PEAR FRUIT

(100 grams = 1 medium fruit)

Calories	40
Fat (grams)	0.5
Cholesterol (milligrams)	0
Carbohydrates (grams)	9.6
Dietary fiber (grams)	3.6
Protein (grams)	0.7
MINERALS	
Calcium (milligrams)	56
Iron (milligrams)	0.3
Magnesium (milligrams)	85
Phosphorus (milligrams)	24
Potassium (milligrams)	220
Sodium (milligrams)	5
Copper (milligrams)	0.08
Selenium (micrograms)	0.6
Zinc (milligrams)	0.12
VITAMINS	
Vitamin C (milligrams)	14
Thiamin (milligrams)	0.01
Riboflavin (milligrams)	0.06
Niacin (milligrams)	0.5
Vitamin B_6 (milligrams)	0.06
Folate (micrograms)	6
Vitamin B_{12} (micrograms)	0
Vitamin A (I.U.)	51
Vitamin E (A.T.E.)	0.01

Source: U.S. Department of Agriculture Nutrient Database

against cancer. Like the pads, the fruit is high in vitamin A in the form of beta-carotene and also vitamin C.

Medicinal Benefits

The fruits of the prickly pear have been under intense scrutiny by researchers in recent years. Scientists have noted positive links between the consumption of the cactus fruit and its antihyperglycemic effects. In a study published by the *International Journal of Pharmacognosy,* researchers found that the daily intake of the prickly pear fruit yielded positive results in laboratory animals. For example, the *Opuntia dillenii* species of the fruit has exhibited a notable antidiabetic effect on rabbits. This species of fruit produced hypoglycemia in rabbits mainly by reducing intestinal absorption of glucose.

Studies at the University of Arizona by Dr. Maria Luz Fernandez, one of the prickly pear's key researchers, show the effects of diet on cholesterol metabolism. Her research includes the use of prickly pear pectin, a glutinous substance found in the cactus fruit. The results of the tests point to a decrease in plasma cholesterol, which is mainly a decrease in low-density lipoprotein.[7] Other results also suggest that prickly pear pectin may modulate the body's glucose response.

CACTUS FLOWERS

In the spring, lovely yellow, orange, or red roselike flowers are produced from the body of the fruit. Like the other two parts of the cactus, the flower petals have been endowed with biologically active compounds that which have medical applications. Similar to rose hips and hibiscus flowers, the cactus flower petals are picked, dried, and then sold in bulk or in tea bags, capsules, or liquid extract.

Vitamin and Mineral Content

If eating or drinking flowers sounds strange, think again. Chances are that you are already consuming flowers in one form or another. Most likely, you are drinking them as a tea. Unknown to many casual tea drinkers, most naturally flavored teas contain hibiscus rose hips for color, taste, and flavonoid content. Not only this, but flower petals are routinely added to multisupplements and antioxidant combinations to buttress the flavonoid content and strengthen the effects of principal antioxidants such as vitamins C and E. Flowers are also commonly sold in the exotic food section of grocery stores. Sprinkling a few flower petals on certain dishes adds some variety, color, and nutrition to what might be an otherwise boring presentation or less nutritious food.

Medicinal Benefits

The cactus flowers are extremely safe to touch and ingest. No toxic or adverse reactions have ever been reported, either for external or internal use. But despite the prickly pear cactus flower's time-honored use, there is little specific scientific information about the flowers. Most of the evidence that supports its use is derived from clinical studies that demonstrate the medicinal effects of the herb's key constituent, the flavonoids.

Recently, scientists have actively explored the employment of the cactus flowers in the treatment of discomforts associated with benign prostatic hypertrophy (BPH), commonly referred to as an enlarged prostate. Clinical studies have indicated a dry flower preparation of the *Opuntia ficus-indica* variety is helpful. Until additional studies are conducted and confirm these same results, prickly pear flowers should not be used as a replacement for other herbal or standard treatments of BPH. For more information refer to the clinical studies in chapter 6 "Other Benefits of and Treatments Using Prickly Pear Cactus."

4

The Cactus-Diabetes Connection

*A study by Alberto C. Frati-Munari and colleagues . . .
published in the January issue of* Diabetes Care *found
that a cactus species used as a food and herbal remedy
in Mexico* (Opuntia Streptacantha), *commonly known
as "Nopal," actually helped lower blood glucose levels
in diabetes patients.*

—Science News[1]

More than twenty years ago, ethnobotanical studies in Mexico identified a group of plants with the highest demand and most frequent use by the Mexican population in the treatment of the symptoms of diabetes.[2] Among these plants was the prickly pear cactus. Its ubiquitous presence as a food among the local cultures throughout the country coupled with its broad array of unique medicinal benefits singled the plant out for research by scientists.

Since that time, the prickly pear has been the subject of research, medicinal studies, and analysis in Mexico and throughout the world. However, it really started with the Mexican scientists' curiosity about the plant that grew in their own backyards. Mexican researchers were curious about the herb's supposed therapeutic value in the treatment of diabetes. They wondered about its effectiveness in treating a number of other ailments as well, including skin and cardiovascular system disorders.

To date, Mexico has assumed a role as the leader in the antidiabetic prickly pear research. This interest has gone on to ignite a global investigation into the prickly pear cactus resulting in recent studies from Europe, the Middle East, and North America. Currently, scientific research involves all three portions of the cactus: pad, fruit, and flower.

This chapter features an aggregate of research from a variety of well-recognized scientific journals published throughout the world. Each study has been effectively summarized, objectively critiqued, and carefully footnoted. These studies examine the hypoglycemic effects of either the prickly pear cactus pads or fruits on animals or humans with classic diabetic symptomology. The studies offer insight into the medicinal effects of several different species of prickly pear cactus, most notably the *Opuntia streptacantha* (to be referred to herein as OS) variety. This species has been the focal point of much antidiabetic herbal research, though additional species of prickly pear are beginning to be recognized for their equally therapeutic effects. Additional varieties of prickly pear that have been the subject of antidiabetic investigation include *Opuntia ficus-indica, Opuntia dillenii,* and *Opuntia fuliginosa.*

Selected portions of these studies may have been excluded from the summaries based on their high level of scientific complexity. An explanation of certain medical concepts is beyond the scope of this book. However, I encourage you to refer to the notes section for a complete bibliographical listing if you are interested in reading the published studies in their entirety.

OPUNTIA STREPTACANTHA

Hypoglycemic Effect of *Opuntia streptacantha* Lemaire in NIDDM *(Diabetes Care)*

Introduction

The purpose of this study was to assess the hypoglycemic effect of *Opuntia streptacantha* (OS) nopal stems on human patients with non-insulin-dependent diabetes mellitus (NIDDM). The research was conducted by a team of scientists from the Mexican Institute of Social Security located in Mexico City. The results of this study were published in January 1998.

The authors note that several previous studies have failed to scientifically validate the antidiabetic medicinal effects of OS. In one such study, the consumption of 100 g of nopal stems did not modify blood sugar levels in humans.[3] However, the authors assert that their study shows that the ingestion of 500 g of OS stems actually does cause a hypoglycemic effect.[4]

Materials and Methods

Three groups of patients were analyzed. Individuals were divided based on the diabetic prescription drug they had been taking over the duration of their illness. Hypoglycemic agents were discontinued seventy-two hours before the study, performed after a twelve-hour fast to purposely raise blood sugar levels. Fresh and tender stems were cleaned and broiled immediately before the experiment.

The study was double blind. One group was chosen to receive fresh extracts of the pad sap while the second, or control group, received an equal volume of water. The purpose of this was to protect the integrity of the study so as not to allow the researchers to indirectly or directly influence the results of the study. The directors of the study, however, were aware of which group received the placebo.

Group 1 received one dose of 500 g of pads. Blood samples were drawn every hour for four hours to measure serum glucose and insulin (at 0, 60, 120, and 180 minutes). Patients in group 2 received only 300 ml of water and blood samples were drawn as in group 1. In group 3, tests with the administration of nopal, water, and a third test with the consumption of squash (as a vegetable substitute for the nopal pads) were implemented in random order, with an interval of at least one week between the tests.

Results

The authors of the study note that previous research has shown that nopal intake can limit the rise of serum glucose after a glucose load, but there was never any observation that nopal intake alone could acutely decrease serum glucose concentrations. This study, however, indicated that the intake of the OS pads actually had a hypoglycemic effect in patients with NIDDM, because a significant decrease of serum glucose value was noticed during the few hours after the nopal intake.

To further understand the results of the studies, it is important to note that milligrams per deciliter (mg/dl) is a unit of measure that shows the concentration of a substance in a specific amount of fluid. In the United States, blood glucose test results are reported as mg/dl. Medical journals and other countries use millimoles per liter (mmol/L). According to the American Diabetes Association, normal fasting blood glucose is below 100 mg/dl. A person with prediabetes has a fasting blood glucose level between 100 and 125 mg/dl. If the blood glucose level rises to 126 mg/dl or above, a person has diabetes.

Basal serum glucose levels of group 1 (221.8 ± 57.8 mg/dl) and group 2 (222.9 ± 57.8 mg/dl) were similar. After consumption of the prickly pear pads (group 1), a decrease in serum glucose levels was noticed at 60 minutes in 12 of the

16 patients. A decrease was later noticed in all patients at 120 and 180 minutes. The decrease in serum glucose concentration was progressive, with a mean ± SE of 19.0 ± 5.4, 23.8 ± 3.3, and 39.1 ± 4.9 mg/dl less than basal value at 60, 120, and 180 minutes, respectively. A decrease in glycemia was also noticed.

In the control subjects, group 2, no changes in serum glucose level or glycemia were noticed with the administration of an amount of water similar to that contained in 500 g of broiled nopal stems. Basal serum insulin concentrations of group 1 also progressively diminished after nopal intake. Serum insulin levels decreased as well. Again, no significant changes were noted in group 2.

In group 3, serum insulin levels significantly decreased after the ingestion of nopal. No similar changes were noted with the control tests. In fact, a slight increase of serum glucose and insulin concentrations occurred after intake of squash. No changes were identified after water intake.

Although there were some patients receiving oral hypoglycemic agents, the influence of a possible residual effect of these drugs on the results should be negligible for two reasons. First, the agents were withdrawn seventy-two hours before the study, and second, a similar proportion of patients receiving the same family of drugs was included in groups 1 and 2. Further, both tests were performed in group 3 and the results of these tests mirrored the results from groups 1 and 2.

Undesirable side effects of OS intake are only an increase in stool volume and frequency and abdominal fullness.

Discussion

The results of this study are in agreement with investigations carried out in diabetic animals, but not with a previous study in which an actual hypoglycemic effect due to nopal ingestion could not be proved.[5] As mentioned earlier, this latter study was performed in healthy subjects who received only 100 g of nopal stems. However, the nopal species was not identified. The pads might not have been of the OS variety.

The scientists postulate several reasons for this difference in results:

1. A hypoglycemic effect appears only in diabetic subjects or only if hyperglycemia is present.
2. A dose of 100 mg of nopal in humans might not be sufficient to elicit a hypoglycemic response. The response might only appear when much higher doses are given.
3. Perhaps only a few species of opuntia cause a hypoglycemic effect.
4. Nopal might have a hypoglycemic effect in addition to a dietary fiber effect. It is worth noting here that dietary fiber is thought to ultimately improve insulin sufficiency. The polysaccharide component (an indigestible carbohydrate) within the cactus is thought to contribute to, through a series of complex chemical reactions, positive changes in glucose and lipid metabolism levels.[6]

The mechanism of action behind the effects of the cactus is unknown. Scientists speculate that the hypoglycemic effect of OS pads may be due to an improvement of glucose cellular utilization. Further, the results of this test suggest that the OS pads contain one or more compounds responsible for the medicinal effects in patients with NIDDM. The article ends with this statement: "These substances or the whole plant stems may be useful in the management of diabetes mellitus."

Opuntia streptacantha:
A Coadjutor in the Treatment of Diabetes Mellitus
(American Journal of Chinese Medicine)

Introduction

This report is a summarization of a research study performed at the biomedical research unit in Traditional Medicine and Herbolary at the Mexican Institute of Social Security, Mexico City, Mexico. A diabetic volunteer was administered a complementary daily dose of OS sap from broiled stems while under treatment with sulfonamides (a synthetic organic bacteria–inhibiting drug). The length of the study was eight weeks.[7]

Materials and Methods

The patient was an obese, fifty-seven-year-old male who had been diagnosed with diabetes mellitus eight years before the study. During this eight-year period, he underwent treatment with a standard prescription drug called chlorpropamide (250 mg per day).

The treatment consisted of an oral dose of 200 ml of OS sap extracted from fresh pads, three times per day before each meal. During the study, the patient continued with his established therapy and his ordinary diet.

Results

The results obtained are shown in table 4.1. The values of glucose and insulin in fasting diminished after treatment with OS pads. The scientists noted a remarkable improvement in the patient's well-being with fewer symptoms than before.

Discussion

The study included only one patient. Under normal circumstances, I would dismiss a study of this sort where the patient

TABLE 4.1
EIGHT WEEK TREATMENT WITH NOPAL PADS

HERB	GLUCOSE mg/dl					INSULIN U/ml				
	Fast	1 hr	2 hr	3 hr	4 hr	Fast	1 hr	2 hr	3 hr	4 hr
CONTROL	204	219	216	187	168	99	124	106	78	79
1	146	182	166	152	124	73	122	98	83	96
2	122	162	160	138	122	36	92	110	91	68
4	118	169	164	164	127	68	106	120	140	116
6	135	200	175	142	137	50	119	94	94	94
8	105	142	137	126	117	38	107	92	98	62

Source: Published in the American Journal of Chinese Medicine, vol. 14, nos. 3–4 (1986): 116–118

sample size does not allow us to accurately draw a strong conclusion. I chose to include this study in the book since the results obtained here corroborate the hypoglycemic effect of OS when it is administered orally to diabetic patients, as displayed in other professional investigations.

Pursuant to the plant's mechanism of action, scientists understand that the hypoglycemic effect could be related to the diminishing of glucose uptake in the intestinal tract absorption. Or it could be related to an increase in the capacity of the insulinic receptors due to the high content of dietary fiber in the stem of this plant.

The scientists suggest that OS fresh sap could be useful as a complementary resource in the treatment of patients with NIDDM. However, additional studies with larger patient sample sizes must be conducted to better understand the effects of complementary therapy. Understanding how complementary therapy works in different gender and age groups is important. Whether gender and age influence the results of complementary therapy is still unconfirmed.

The Hypoglycemic Effect of *Opuntia streptacantha* Studied in Different Animal Experimental Models (*Journal of Ethnopharmacology*)

Introduction

Scientists from Mexico's biomedical research unit at the Mexican Institute of Social Security in Mexico City performed studies with the sap of fresh prickly pear cactus pads (OS) in three different animal species to determine the plant's antidiabetic effects.[8]

Materials and Methods

Success with earlier studies conducted with the fresh extract of OS stems and its therapeutic effect on animal blood sugar levels drove the same group of scientists to conduct an additional study on the effects of the cactus pads. Here, the studies were performed with the same fresh extract of cactus pads in three different animal species under various experimental conditions. The three animal species utilized in the study were rats, rabbits, and dogs.

In all cases, before the start of the studies, the animals were submitted to an eighteen-hour fasting period. Studies performed were double blind. Several different experimental conditions were chosen. For example, animals were administered OS sap in either awake or anesthetized states. Some were administered the sap after a period of fasting; others after being administered an intravenous glucose load to artificially raise glucose levels in the blood.

Stocks of 1.0 kg of fresh OS stems were used. The stems were melted without water and the sap obtained (500 ml) was carefully filtered. The filtered sap was then orally administered to the animals in a 5.0 ml/kg body weight dose by means of a plastic probe. Blood samples were then obtained several times during the length of the study and mean blood glucose levels were compared.

Results

The results indicate that the cactus sap induced hypoglycemic effects when orally administered to animals under induced states of moderate increase of blood sugar. The results of this study validated the popular use of the herb for the treatment of diabetes mellitus symptomology.[9] No changes in blood sugar level were detected in animals with normal levels of blood sugar.

Discussion

The authors comment that it is difficult to create a perfect study of the OS sap or any other hypoglycemic drugs because experimental diabetes induced in animals is not exactly the same as the pathological condition observed in patients. Second, the scientists called for additional analytical chemical studies to identify the active compounds present in the cactus pad sap. Due to a lack of available published analysis of biologically active agents in the prickly pear at the time of the study, the scientists were not fully capable of identifying the mechanism of action behind the plant's hypoglycemic effect.

Antihyperglycemic Effect of Some Edible Plants (*Journal of Ethnopharamacology*)

Introduction

The objective of this study was to research the potential antihyperglycemic effect of 12 edible plants. The double-blind study was performed on 27 healthy rabbits. Included on the list of edible plants was OS.[10]

Materials and Methods

The fasting animals were split into three groups. The first group, the control group, was given a subcutaneous glucose tolerance test after gastric administration of water. The second group, the reference control group, was administered tolbutamide, a medication used in the treatment of non-insulin-dependent diabetes. The experimental group received the traditional preparation of the OS plant. Blood glucose levels were measured in fasting and at one-hour intervals for five hours.

Results

The extract demonstrated a significant decrease in blood glucose values as demonstrated by a decrease of 17.8 percent in the area under the glucose tolerance curve and a decrease of 18 percent in the hyperglycemic peak as compared to controls.

Discussion

Positive results of the study led the researchers to conclude that future possibilities might allow diabetic patients to reduce their dosages of current hypoglycemic agents by incorporating plants into their diet. The obvious and unique benefit of plants such as the OS is that they function as both food and medicine. Results of this study show that patients with mild type II diabetes can possibly avoid the use of prescription hypoglycemic agents and control blood glucose through diet and/or nutritional supplementation alone.

Influence of Nopal Intake upon Fasting Glycemia in Type II Diabetics and Healthy Subjects (*Medical Investigation Archives*)

Introduction

The purpose of the test was to assess whether the acute hypoglycemic effect of the OS pads that occurs in diabetic patients also occurs in healthy individuals. This study was conducted by Alberto Frati, one of the leaders in the field of investigation into the therapeutic benefits of the prickly pear. The study was published in 1991.[11]

Materials and Methods

500 g of nopal stems were given orally to 14 healthy volunteers and to 14 patients diagnosed with NIDDM. Serum glucose and insulin levels were to be measured at the start of the study, and every 60 minutes thereafter for three hours. A control test group was to receive an equivalent amount of water.

Results

The NIDDM group responded positively to the effects of the cactus and exhibited a significant reduction of serum glucose and insulin concentration reaching 40.8 ± 4.6 mg/dl and 7.8 ± 1.5 µU/ml less than baseline value, at 180 minutes. No significant changes were noticed in the healthy group as compared with the control test group. Note: Unit of Insulin (U) is the basic measure of insulin. U-100 insulin means 100 units of insulin per milliliter (ml) or cubic centimeter (cc) of solution.

Discussion

Since no hypoglycemic change was noted in the healthy control group but only in the NIDDM group, it appears that the effects of the OS pads are hyperglycemic specific. In other words, the OS pads are only therapeutically beneficial in individuals who display high blood sugar levels.

More on *Opuntia streptacantha*

In order to avoid repeating information already documented in this chapter, the following list provides information culled from additional test studies on the use of the OS pads for the treatment of diabetic symptomology.

- The consumption of OS stems before meals for 10 days was followed by a mean decrease of 63.4 mg/dl in blood glucose levels.[12]

- The ingestion of OS stems was found to diminish the rise of blood glucose levels that follows a dextrose load in humans and in experimental animals.[13]

- No seasonal variation in the hypoglycemic activity of the OS stems was detected. This suggests that the plants can be harvested and utilized year-round for the treatment of diabetes mellitus.[14]

- A second repeated dose of OS stems two hours after the first dose did not improve the herb's hypoglycemic activity. A progressive drop in serum glucose levels was noted due to the first dose. However, there was no marked change as a result of an additional dose. [15]

- Scientists in this study recognized a significant correlation between the ingestion of OS pads and a hypoglycemic effect. Their lack of understanding of the mechanism of action behind the dose's effect, however, did not allow the scientists to verify a causal effect.[16]

- The hypoglycemic activity of ingested OS pads is progressive and became more pronounced by the fourth hour. No significant change was noted from the fourth to the sixth hour after initial administration of cactus. In this study, 500 g of OS pads were broiled and ingested.[17]

- Additional research confirms the finding that the hypoglycemic activity of OS pads is hyperglycemic specific. In other words, there is no hypoglycemic effect in healthy individuals, unless hyperglycemia is present in healthy persons. In this test, healthy volunteers ingested 500 g of broiled OS pads.[18]

- This research study focused on the potential healthful effects of the crude raw version of the herb versus cooked. 500 g of OS stems were utilized. The intake of broiled OS stems caused a significant decrease of serum glucose level that reached 48.3 ± 16.2 mg/dl lower than baseline values (after 180 minutes). The raw extract failed to create a significant decrease of glycemia. As it has been recorded in other studies, it appears that the heating of the OS pads is necessary to obtain the hypoglycemic effect. [19]

OPUNTIA FICUS-INDICA

Effect of a Dehydrated Extract of Nopal *(Opuntia ficus-indica)* (OFI) on Blood Glucose *(Medical Investigation Archives)*

Introduction

The purpose of the following study was to assess whether a dehydrated extract of OFI stems retains any therapeutic effect on glycemia. The study was conducted by researchers in Mexico.[20]

Materials and Methods

Two double-blind studies were performed. The first study was comprised of six patients with type II diabetes mellitus. After fasting, each patient received 30 capsules containing 10.1 ± 0.3 g of OFI stem extract. Their serum glucose levels were measured hourly for three hours, including during administration. The second group, the control, received empty capsules.

The second test was made up of six healthy volunteers who received 30 capsules of the OFI stem extract followed by the oral administration of 74 g of dextrose. Serum glucose measurements were conducted in a similar fashion to the first test. A control group also received 30 empty capsules.

Results

The results of the test were negative. The OFI extract did not reduce fasting glycemia in diabetic subjects. Nevertheless, the extract diminished the increase of serum glucose, which followed a dextrose load. Peak serum glucose was 20.3 ± 18.2 mg/dl lower in the test with nopal than in the control group.

The scientists concluded that the dehydrated extract of OFI did not show acute hypoglycemic effect. No changes were noted in the healthy subjects.

Discussion

Because the preparation of the crude extract lost some of its hypoglycemic action, the authors hypothesized that heating the extracts or the entire stems prior to administration might be necessary in order to elicit the antidiabetic effect. Later studies by these scientists explored the use of crude versus broiled OFI in the treatment of diabetic symptomology. As you will see in the following study, certain preparations of the crude OFI are effective. The methods of preparation are as integral to the healing process as is the method of administration.

Hypoglycemic Effect of *Opuntia ficus-indica* in Non-Insulin-Dependent Diabetes Mellitus Patients *(Phytotherapy Research)*

Introduction

The purpose of this study was to assess whether the prickly pear stems, or their crude or heated preparations, from the OFI variety, demonstrate a hypoglycemic effect in patients with NIDDM. The majority of research with the prickly pear cactus has been with the OS variety. Yet the OS variety is less palatable than the OFI species. The latter species is commonly sold and used as a food source for people in Mexico; however, its hypoglycemic effect has not been established. The research was carried out by researchers at the Department of Internal Medicine at the Mexican Institute of Social Security in Mexico City, Mexico.[21]

Materials and Methods

Eight NIDDM patients, six females and two males, were studied. Their ages ranged from forty-five to sixty-eight years. Diabetes had been diagnosed an average of 11.5 years before entry to the study.

OFI stems were collected and kept refrigerated for one to three weeks until the test was performed. The day before the study, the stems were washed and thorns and some cuticle were removed. Five separate tests were conducted preparing the OFI for administration in different ways. Each test was performed as follows:

1. *Entire broiled stems:* The entire stems were broiled on a conventional grill and cut in 2 to 3 cm pieces.
2. *Blended broiled stems:* After the stems were broiled, they were chopped in a conventional blender for 2 minutes.
3. *Blended crude stems:* Similar to test 2 but with crude stems.
4. *Heated blended stems:* After blending, crude fractions were heated at 60° C/140° F for 10 minutes before ingestion
5. *Double-blind control test:* Performed with 400 ml of water instead of OFI extracts.

Each test was performed on all eight patients in a random order with an interval of at least seventy-two hours between tests. Hypoglycemic agents were discontinued three days prior to each test. All the tests were carried out in the morning with a twelve-hour overnight fast. A blood sample was obtained (0 minutes) followed immediately by ingestion of OFI or placebo. Then serial venous blood samples were taken at 30, 60, 120, and 180 minutes.

Results

Basal serum glucose levels were similar in the five tests performed. A decrease in glycemia levels was noticed with entire broiled stems of OFI as well as with different crude and broiled blended preparations. Glycemia values were significantly lower than those obtained in the control test. The maximal decrease observed in the serum glucose levels after OFI administration ranged from 22.3 ± 4.4 to 25.3 ± 14.3 mg/dl below those obtained at 0 minutes. There were no significant decreases noticed between heated and unheated crude preparations of OFI.

Discussion

The hypoglycemic effect elicited by OFI in this study seems to be unrelated to dietary fiber mechanisms (for example, changes in the intestinal absorption of glucose), since patients did not receive an oral dextrose load before the OFI preparations were administered.

Here too the researchers cite that the precise mechanism of action behind OFI is unknown, as it is for OS. It was originally thought by researchers that heating the stems could be necessary in order to exert its hypoglycemic effect. However, the fact that blended crude and cold OFI stems showed the same activity as that of the heated preparations used in this study lends no further support to this hypothesis.

Differences between these investigations might be better explained by the procedure of homogenation; in the former study, the researchers think that ultrahomogenation probably disrupted the structure of proteins or other substances, while a conventional blender, as used in this study, did not.

Evaluation of Nopal Capsules in Diabetes Mellitus (*Gaceta Medica de Mexico*)

Introduction

The same group of researchers who prepared the above study on the effects of the administration of OFI on diabetes mellitus symptomology also prepared this study. The objective was to determine if commercial capsules prepared with dried OFI stems play a role in the management of diabetes mellitus.[22]

Materials and Methods

Three separate experiments were performed. The first double-blind study involved 10 diabetic patients in fasting condition who were administered 30 capsules of dried nopal. Their serum glucose levels were measured throughout the next three hours following consumption of the cactus. Group 2, the control group, received 30 placebo capsules. Their serum glucose levels were monitored the same as group 1.

The second double-blind study was made up of 10 healthy individuals who did not display diabetic symptomology. Two groups were created: one group to receive the nopal and the other group to receive placebo capsules. The scientists monitored serum glucose levels.

The next study was a crossover and single-blind study in which 14 diabetic patients received either 10 nopal or placebo capsules three times per day for one week. Serum glucose, cholesterol, and triglyceride levels were measured before and after each one-week period. Five healthy subjects were also studied in the same fashion.

Results

OFI capsules failed to show acute hypoglycemic effect. In diabetic patients in study 1, serum glucose, cholesterol, and triglyceride levels did not significantly change. The healthy individuals' (the subjects of study 2) serum glucose levels did not change, while their cholesterol and triglyceride levels decreased.

Discussion

The effect on glucose and cholesterol that the OFI capsules had on the diabetic individuals was discretely beneficial. However, the authors of the study acknowledge that the dose is impractical and recommend against the use of OFI capsules to treat diabetes.

Currently, there are several companies in the natural products industry who encapsulate dried OFI stems for the purposes of maintaining blood sugar levels. While the ingestion of crude or broiled OFI stems has proven to be beneficial, there is currently debate on whether the encapsulated form shares this same healthful effect. The results of this study state that the latter may not be the case. One research study, however, does not provide enough of a base to dismiss the potential effectiveness of OFI capsules in the treatment of hyperglycemia. There may be variables present in this study that negatively influenced the results of the test, such as quality and presence of active components in OFI or drying methods.

As additional studies are required to determine the surety of the utilization of encapsulated OFI in the management of diabetes mellitus, it is not recommended as a preferred treatment.

OPUNTIA FULIGINOSA

A Purified Extract from Prickly Pear Cactus (*Opuntia fuliginosa*) Controls Experimentally Induced Diabetes in Rats
(*Journal of Ethnopharamcology*)

Introduction

The purpose of the study was to evaluate the hypoglycemic activity of a purified extract from the prickly pear cactus fruit, utilizing the *Opuntia fuliginosa* (OF) variety. The experiment evaluated the plant's ability to control experimentally induced diabetes in rats. Diabetes was induced by intraperitoneal injection of streptozotocin (STZ). The authors of the study are based out of the Department of Biotechnology in the state of Michoacán, Mexico. The study was published in 1996.[23]

Materials and Methods

The first group was to receive only OF extract. The second group, induced with diabetes, was to be treated with insulin alone. The third group of diabetes-induced rats was administered both OF and insulin as a combined treatment. As part of this portion of the study, insulin was withdrawn from the combined treatment to examine whether or not the prickly pear cactus could alone maintain a normoglycemic state in the diabetic rats. The glucose levels of the fourth group, the nondiabetic control group, were to be monitored throughout the experiment. The OF extract was administered daily through a gastric catheter.

Results

The first and second groups, the rats receiving only OF extract, had glucose levels similar to those of insulin-treated rats. In the third group, blood glucose and glycated hemoglobin levels were reduced to normal values by a combined treatment of insulin and OF extract. When insulin was withdrawn from the combined treatment in week eight, due to hypoglycemia, the OF extract successfully maintained normoglycemic state in the rats. The blood glucose response to administered glucose also showed that those receiving the combination treatment of insulin and OF extract for seven weeks followed by OF alone were capable of rapidly returning blood glucose to the levels of the nondiabetic rats. The glucose levels of the nondiabetic control group remained similar to initial levels.

Discussion

The mechanism of action was not identified by the authors, but the authors conclude that dietary fiber probably plays a predominant role. The authors cite the results of this study as very encouraging and believe these positive results for diabetes control by the purified extract of OF make the need for clinical studies in humans more evident.

The important take-away from this study is that the control of diabetes by purified extract of opuntia can be attained with daily oral doses in the range of 1 mg/kg body weight.

A Note on *O. fuliginosa* Fruit

Dr. Augusta Trejo, while at the National Polytechnic Institute in Michoacán, Mexico, conducted a number of different experiments with prickly pear fruit pectin and people with diabetes. Dr. Trejo found that by giving 60 mg (about the size of one drop from an eyedropper) a day of prickly pear pectin, the diabetics were able to significantly lower their insulin requirement. Other types of pectin brought about the same result but were required in much higher amounts—on the order of 15 to 20 g per day.[24]

OPUNTIA DILLENII

Antihyperglycemic Effect of Fresh *Opuntia dillenii* Fruit from Tenerife (Canary Islands)
(International Journal of Pharmacognosy)

Introduction

The fresh fruit of the prickly pear cactus, *Opuntia dillenii* (OD), is used as an antidiabetic agent in Canary Islands folk medicine. To determine whether or not there is a scientific basis for this popular use, the effects of the fruit's red palatable juice on blood glucose levels were assessed in normoglycemic and alloxan-induced diabetic rabbits. The scientists also assessed the fruit for toxicity in rats. The tests were conducted at the Institute of Pharmacology and Department of Cellular Biology at the University of Camerino in Italy.[25]

Materials and Methods

OD was collected in the month of June. The fresh fruit was crushed without using water. The palatable, dense red juice obtained was filtered and then frozen until use.

Male rabbits were employed in the study. Diabetes mellitus was introduced by a single injection of the drug alloxan after the rabbits had been subjected to an overnight fast to determine glycemia values at zero time (start of study). The control group received an equivalent volume of distilled water. They then rested for one week to allow the diabetes to develop and reach a steady state. For the toxicity test, healthy adult male rats were used.

EXPERIMENT 1

The purpose of the first experiment was to assess OD for toxicity in rats. Sixty-four rats were divided into eight groups of 8. Groups 1 to 4 received OD juice in single doses; groups 5 to 8 received equivalent volumes of distilled water. The rats were observed for eight hours after each dosing to check for toxicity and were kept under observation for seven days.

The second part of the experiment involved treating two groups of seven rats with daily does of OD juice for seven days. The two control groups received equivalent volumes of water.

EXPERIMENT 2

The purpose of the second experiment was to determine the effect of OD juice on blood glucose levels of normoglycemic and diabetic-induced rabbits. The first two groups of normoglycemic and diabetic rabbits received a single dose (5 ml/kg) of juice. Their respective control groups received the equivalent amount of distilled water. Blood samples were collected at the beginning of the study and every thirty minutes for up to four hours following dosing.

In the second half of the experiment, two additional groups of normoglycemic and diabetic-induced rabbits received 5 mg/kg juice daily for seven days. The control groups received an equal amount of water. All rabbits were fasted overnight. On the eighth day another load of juice or water was administered. Blood samples were collected at the start of the study at zero time and every 30 minutes for four hours on the eighth day.

EXPERIMENT 3

Normoglyemic and diabetic rabbits received OD juice (5 ml/kg); one hour later they received glucose. The control group received an initial administration of water followed by an equivalent amount of glucose. Blood samples were monitored as they were in experiment 2.

In the second part of the study, another group of fasted normoglycemic rabbits received a glucose solution (1 g/kg) 60 minutes after oral administration of 5 ml/kg of the OD juice. A control group received 5 ml/kg of water, and 60 minutes later received intravenously (IV) 1 g/kg glucose. Blood glucose concentrations were determined at zero time, prior to juice or water oral load, and at every 30 minutes for up to three hours following IV glucose load.

EXPERIMENT 4

The chief purpose of this study was to compare the hypoglycemic effect of OD with that of tolbutamide, a clinically used antidiabetic drug. A single oral dose of the prescription drug (100 mg/kg suspended in a 5 ml volume) was assessed under identical conditions of oral glucose load as described in the first part of experiment three. The control groups received 5 percent gum arabic suspension.

Results

The results of the four experiments are as follows:

EXPERIMENT 1

In the acute toxicity test, all rats given single doses of OD appeared normal. No symptoms indicating toxicity were seen.

In the subacute toxicity test, the rats dosed with 5 or 10 ml/kg for seven days also appeared healthy and active for the entire observation period. None of the rats died.

EXPERIMENT 2

The blood glucose levels following a single oral dose of juice did not differ significantly between control and treated groups of either normoglycemic or alloxan-induced diabetic rabbits. The glucose values at the different times after treatment were strictly similar to those determined at zero time.

In the second part of the experiment, the repeated oral doses of juice were also completely ineffective in either normo-glycemic or alloxan-induced diabetic rabbits.

EXPERIMENT 3

In this experiment, the crude drug markedly reduced the pro-gressively elevated glucose values, and the effect was statisti-cally significant for the entire three-hour period of observation. The overall analysis of variance revealed a marked treatment effect.

OD in juice form also reduced glucose-induced hyper-glycemia in the alloxan-induced diabetic rabbits. The analysis of variance revealed a significant treatment effect and treat-ment time interaction.

EXPERIMENT 4

As expected by the scientists, tolbutamide produced a significant effect in normoglycemic rabbits orally loaded with glucose. It did not produce this same effect in alloxan-induced diabetic rabbits. This finding agrees with the drug's mechanism of action.

Discussion

The drug reduced the progressive increase of blood glucose levels in normoglycemic rabbits and in alloxan-induced diabetic rabbits. The antihyperglycemic effect was pronounced, especially in the normoglycemic animals, and long lasting.

The scientists concluded that the OD juice may reduce the intestinal absorption of glucose. Its mechanism of action, they hypothesize, may be due to an orally active insulin-like compound, as reported in other studies on species of prickly pear. (It should be noted that when the glucose load was administered intravenously, the fruit juice was ineffective; when it was administered orally, on the other hand, it was effective.)

The results of this study show that OD fruit possesses active constituents capable of lowering blood glucose levels. This effect noticed in the lab provides scientific basis for the historic use of this drug. Given this effect and the herb's low toxicity, this fruit could be very helpful in reducing the dangerous hyperglycemia induced by the ingestion of large amounts of carbohydrates, without producing any hypoglycemic effect under normal conditions.

The researchers also state that the herb could be used in treatment when administered simultaneously with another hypoglycemic agent to diabetic patients, as previously demonstrated in other studies with the use of OS stems. The scientists recognize that further comprehensive clinical and pharmacological investigations are necessary to identify the exact mechanism of action behind the fruit's antidiabetic effect. Additional studies are also needed to determine the long-term effects of treatment with this crude herb.

TOXICITY

None of the clinical trials on either the prickly pear pads or fruits showed that consumption of the three species here (OS, OFI, and OD) exert any side effects or aftereffects in terms of toxicity. Large numbers of people have consumed both the pads and fruits for many years without reports of toxicity. However, consuming the fresh pads without properly scrubbing them and removing the thorns may result in a severely unpleasant chewing experience.

The Cactus-Cholesterol Connection

If you have high cholesterol, here is some new advice:
eat more prickly pear.
—Arizona Daily Star[1]

An impressive number of high-quality studies have been carried out on the prickly pear cactus and its effect on cholesterol metabolism. The research performed on the cactus-cholesterol connection has largely focused on the use of the fruit as medicine. Its compounds, which include antioxidants and pectin, have made it a popular subject of cholesterol test studies. This chapter contains an amalgam of those studies. As in the previous chapter, each of the studies listed has been analyzed, critiqued, and footnoted. Selected portions of these studies may have been excluded from the summaries based on their high level of scientific complexity. An explanation of certain medical concepts is beyond the scope of the book. Yet I encourage you to refer to the notes for a complete citation if you are interested in reading the published studies in their entirety.

WHAT IS PECTIN?

Scientists today have postulated that the role of dietary soluble fiber in human health has potentially beneficial effects in decreasing plasma cholesterol concentrations and in delaying glucose absorption.[2] Their research includes a variety of fibers including pectin. Pectin, as one of the predominant components of dietary fiber, has been the focal point of much research.

Much of the investigation on the prickly pear cactus fruit starts with pectin. After all, it is a main biological constituent of the prickly pear fruit. But the soluble fiber credited with modulating glucose response and reducing plasma cholesterol levels exists in a lot of other fruits and vegetables as well, including apples, bananas, beans, carrots, cherries, grapes, grapefruits, kiwi fruits, lemons, oranges, sugar beet pulp, sunflower heads, and sweet potatoes. The levels of pectin concentration vary for these different plant tissues, however, and not all pectin is created equal. Recent research included in this chapter sheds light on the special qualities of prickly pear fruit pectin. It appears that the high-fiber, gelatinous substance from the fruit of the cactus is especially potent. True to its potential, it is seemingly more potent than pectin from other sources, making it increasingly popular as a cholesterol-lowering food.

OPUNTIA STREPTACANTHA FRUIT

Prickly Pear *(Opuntia sp.)* Pectin Alters Hepatic Cholesterol Metabolism without Affecting Cholesterol Absorption in Guinea Pigs* Fed a Hypercholesterolemic Diet *(Journal of Nutrition)*

Introduction

Various dietary soluble fibers, including pectin, guar gum, psyllium, and oat bran, have been shown to decrease plasma cho-

---

*All animal experiments were conducted in accordance with U.S. Public Health Service and U.S. Department of Agriculture guidelines, and experimental protocols were approved by the University of Arizona Institutional Animal Care and Use Committee.

lesterol levels in humans and several animal species. The specific effects, however, of soluble fiber on cholesterol absorption and hepatic cholesterol homeostasis vary, depending on the experimental design, the animal model, and the soluble fiber tested. The purpose of this study was to investigate whether prickly pear pectin (derived from the fruit) has an effect on cholesterol absorption and on enzymes responsible for cholesterol homeostasis. The study was conducted at the Department of Nutritional Sciences and Interdisciplinary Nutritional Sciences Program at the University of Arizona. The study was supported in part by a grant-in-aid from the American Heart Association, Arizona Affiliate.[3]

Materials and Methods

Male guinea pigs weighing 250 to 300 g were randomly assigned to one of three dietary groups. After week four, the animals were killed by anesthetization and subsequently examined to obtain liver and plasma for isolation of hepatic microsomes and plasma lipoproteins. All animals consumed equal amounts of diet. All diets contained 15 g of lard per 100 g diet. The three diets consisted of:

1. The lard-basal diet with no added cholesterol or prickly pear pectin (LB diet)
2. The LB diet with 0.25 g added cholesterol per 100 g diet (LC diet)
3. The LC diet containing 2.5 g prickly pear pectin per 100 g diet added at the expense of cellulose (LC-P diet)

Next, several tools of analysis, which included the determination of total plasma cholesterol and a hepatic enzyme assay, were conducted.

Note: Guinea pigs were chosen in this and other studies as the experimental animal model because of their similarities to humans in terms of the plasma lipoprotein profile. The reasons here include the distribution of the hepatic free and esterified cholesterol pools, and the relative activities of the hepatic enzymes. In short, like humans, guinea pigs have high levels of LDL relative to levels of HDL. Further, guinea pigs also have a tissue distribution of whole body cholesterol synthesis similar to that of humans.[4]

Results

Animals fed the LB diet (*without* added cholesterol and prickly pear cactus pectin) had the lowest plasma LDL and hepatic cholesterol concentrations, followed by animals fed the LC-P diet. Plasma LDL cholesterol concentrations were 31 percent lower in the group fed the LC-P diet compared with values for the LC diet–fed group. The plasma cholesterol lowering was specific to LDL, because plasma VLDL and HDL cholesterol concentrations were unaffected.

Hepatic free and esterified cholesterol concentrations were lowest in animals fed the LB diet. Intake of cholesterol (LC diet) resulted in higher hepatic cholesterol concentrations, and intake of prickly pear pectin partially lowered these values. Compared with values for animals fed the LC diet, hepatic free and esterified cholesterol concentrations were reduced in animals fed the LC-P diet by 18 percent and 57 percent respectively. No side- or after-effects were documented in the study.

Discussion

The authors of the study confirm that the intake of prickly pear pectin does lower hepatic cholesterol concentration, resulting in effects on hepatic cholesterol homeostasis and on plasma LDL concentrations. The primary mechanism by which these metabolic changes occur is still unknown.

It is thought that one possible mechanism by which prickly pear could have a hypocholesterolemic effect would be its ability to bind bile acids, which would reduce hepatic cholesterol concentration by increasing the demand for hepatic cholesterol. In fact, previous research studies using pectin in humans and rats have found that it reduces cholesterol absorption. However, these studies used higher concentrations of pectin than were used in the present study (2.5 g/100 g diet). Another mechanism by which the prickly pear pectin could have a hypocholesterolemic effect is by production of short-chain fatty acids resulting from fermentation of the fiber in the colon.

The authors' results also point to a peculiar effect of prickly pear pectin. They assert that intake of cactus fruit pectin at 2.5 g per 100 g diet demonstrates the same effect as citrus pectin intake of 7.5 to 10.0 g/100 g diet. This data suggests that these two sources of dietary pectin result in different dose-response effects on hepatic cholesterol homeostasis.

Pectin Isolated from Prickly Pear *(Opuntia sp.)* Modifies Low-Density Lipoprotein Metabolism in Cholesterol-Fed Guinea Pigs *(Journal of Nutrition)*

Introduction

Dietary fiber has been reported to reduce plasma cholesterol levels by binding to bile acids and increasing bile acid fecal excretion. However, the type and amount of dietary fiber and the presence of other nutrients in the diet influence the biochemical properties of fiber and its effect on cholesterol and lipoprotein metabolism. The objective of the study was to examine the effect of prickly pear soluble fiber on low-density lipoprotein (LDL) metabolism. Since this pectin has been used successfully to treat diabetic patients at concentrations as low as 60 mg/day, the effect on LDL metabolism was investigated.

These studies were conducted at the University of Arizona (UofA) supported in part by a grant-in-aid from the American

Heart Association, Arizona Affiliate, a grant from the National Dairy Council, and funds provided by UofA.[5]

Materials and Methods

Male guinea pigs were randomly assigned to one of two diets. Both diets were prepared from a single batch diet that contained 0.25 percent added recrystalized cholesterol. The diets were differentiated by the addition of 1.0 percent prickly pear pectin:

1. Had no added prickly pear pectin (HC diet)
2. The HC diet with 1.0 percent added prickly pear pectin (HC-P diet)

A process called enzymatic analysis determined total plasma cholesterol and triglyceride levels. This included examination of cholesterol content of liver and of plasma total, VLDL, LDL, and HDL cholesterol levels.

Results

The HC-P diet–fed group exhibited a significant 26 percent reduction in plasma total cholesterol levels as compared to levels in animals fed the HC diet. Triglyceride levels did not differ between animals fed the two diets.

A significant percent decrease in plasma LDL and HDL cholesterol levels was observed in HC-P–fed guinea pigs. VLDL cholesterol concentrations were elevated in guinea pigs fed the HC-P diet, although not significantly. Also, the researchers noted that some guinea pigs had a more pronounced response than others did to prickly pear pectin in the presence of the high-cholesterol diet. On average, an overall 26 percent reduction in total cholesterol and 33 percent reduction in LDL and HDL cholesterol were observed.

The addition of pectin to diets results in a decrease in liver cholesterol content, as reported by many investigators. In these studies, the researchers noted that a similar response was observed in that prickly pear pectin significantly reduced hepatic total, free, and esterified cholesterol levels when compared with levels with the HC diet.

Hepatic concentrations of total, free, and esterified cholesterol were significantly reduced in guinea pigs fed the HC-P diet by 85 percent. This is compared with a 40 percent decrease in the animals fed the HC diet. No side- or aftereffects were documented in the study. See table 5.1 for a summary of the plasma lipid results in guinea pigs in this study.

Discussion

The authors report that "pectin from various sources, including citrus pectin and other commercial brands, has been consistently found to reduce plasma cholesterol levels in animal models when fed at levels ranging from 5 to 20 percent. This cholesterol-lowering effect has been observed even in the presence of high fat and high cholesterol diets. In clinical studies, pectin has also shown a hypocholesterolemic effect in normal and hyperlipidemic subjects."[6]

The researchers subsequently determined that prickly pear

TABLE 5.1
PLASMA LIPIDS IN GUINEA PIGS

PLASMA LIPIDS	DIET	
	HC	HC-P
	mg/100mL	
Total Cholesterol	89 +/- 24	66 +/- 29
Total Triglycerides	54 +/- 14	52 +/- 23
Lipoprotein Cholesterol		
High-Density Lipoprotein	5 +/- 2	10 +/- 12
Low-Density Liprotein	59 +/- 24	39 +/- 15
Very Low-Density Liprotein	22 +/- 7	15 +/- 5

Source: "Pectin Isolated from Prickly Pear (Opuntia sp.) Modifies Low-Density Lipoprotein Metabolism in Cholesterol-Fed Guinea Pigs." The Journal of Nutrition, vol. 120 (1990).

pectin had a hypocholesterolemic effect that affected both LDL and HDL fractions when fed at a concentration as low as 1.0 percent. In the present study, adding pectin to the HC diet resulted in normalization of plasma LDL and HDL cholesterol levels.

Because pectin was added to the HC diet at a concentration of only 1.0 percent, it would be of interest to determine the hypocholesterolemic response to prickly pear pectin when fed at higher concentrations of 5 to 15 percent, as used for studies of other fibers by various investigators. More studies utilizing higher concentrations are needed to better assess the dose-response to gauge a potentially higher level of effectiveness and a faster treatment period.

Regarding the proposed mechanism of action, the authors conclude that the mechanisms involved in the plasma hypocholesterolemic effect of the cactus pectin could be analogous to those reported for the prescription drug cholestyramine and other bile acid–binding resins in clinical and animal studies.

More on *Opuntia streptacantha*

- Previous studies in guinea pigs have shown that intake of pectin isolated from prickly pear by animals fed a hypercholesterolemic diet results in a significant decrease in plasma LDL cholesterol due to increased hepatic apolipoprotein B/E receptor expression and receptor-mediated LDL catabolism.[7]
- LDL composition was modified by intake of cactus pectin. An increase in apolipoprotein B/E receptor expression is a major metabolic response by which intake of prickly pear pectin decreases plasma LDL concentrations. [8]

OPUNTIA DILLENII FRUIT

Effects of Cactus and Ginger Extracts as Dietary Antioxidants on Reactive Oxidant and Plasma Lipid Level *(Food Science Biotechnology)*

Introduction

Many scientists have suggested that dietary antioxidants such as ascorbate, tocopherol, and carotenoids from fruits and vegetables could help to protect cells from damage caused by oxidative stress and fortify the defense systems against degenerative diseases.[9] The authors note that the prickly pear cactus fruit has been used as a source of carbohydrates and vitamins for a long time in several countries and was utilized as a jam, jelly, and juice in Mexico and Japan. Moreover, it is known that the cactus (Opuntia dillenii; OD) grown on Jeju Island contains phenolic compounds and flavonoids as major components. These compounds possess particular abilities as anticarcinogens, antioxidants, detoxificants, and antimutagens.[10]

Aware of research on the cactus for the purpose of antioxidant usage and its beneficial effect on blood lipids, the scientists in this study looked to further evaluate the role of the cactus extract as medicine. The study was carried out to investigate the effects of water or ethanol extracts of cactus against reactive antioxidants, and on lipid levels in mouse plasma. The test studies were performed at the Chonnam National University in Korea.[11]

Materials and Methods

Samples of OD were obtained from local markets at Young-am kun in Chonnam, Korea, and Jeju Island. Two types of cactus extracts were created: a cactus water extract (CWE) and a cactus ethanol extract (CEA).

Mice, aged forty-five to fifty weeks, were divided into five groups with 6 mice per group (control, water, or ethanol extracts from cactus and ginger). Mice were administered orally at dose of 600 mg/kg once a day for 10 days. On day 11, blood was collected.

To investigate the effect of the cactus extracts on lipid levels in mouse plasma, the amounts of TG, TC, HDL, LDL, and VLDL (triglyceride, total plasma cholesterol, high-density lipoprotein, low-density lipoprotein, and very low-density lipoprotein) were measured.

Next, the blood was screened, utilizing four separate assays, for its antioxidative activity. The tests were performed at a 95 percent confidence interval (a set of values used to estimate the true value of an experimental variable).

Results

In the first assay, both extracts of cactus were estimated to have antioxidative ability as protectors of reactive oxidants. Among the extracts, the CWE, prepared with distilled water, was shown to have more scavenging activities than the cactus extract with ethanolic solvent. It should be noted that from the results of the study, it was found that the scavenging activities of cactus extracts against hydroxy radicals were more than in ginger extracts, while those against superoxide were similar among all extracts.

Pursuant to the cholesterol assays, in treatment of cactus extracts, the amount of TC, TG, LDL, and VLDL were reduced significantly, while those in ginger extracts were not decreased statistically. In the case of HDL, the amount was not increased by treatment of cactus extracts, compared with that of control mice. Refer to table 5.2 for effects of the cactus extract on plasma cholesterol levels in mice, compared to the control.

As shown in table 5.2, the amounts of TC, TG, LDL, and VLDL in mouse plasma were reduced considerably in the groups treated with cactus extracts, compared to the control.

TABLE 5.2. EFFECTS OF CACTUS EXTRACT PLASMA
CHOLESTEROL LEVELS IN MICE

CHOLESTEROLS (mg/dl)	CONTROL	CACTUS (OD)	
		WATER EXTRACT	ETHANOL EXTRACT
Triglycerides	130.80 +/- 5.67	113.40 +/- 7.83	116.80 +/- 5.72
Total Plasma Cholesterol	197.60 +/- 3.05	186.80 +/- 6.05	187.60 +/- 3.51
High-Density Lipoprotein	35.40 +/- 4.04	40.0 +/- 1.58	41.40 +/- 2.07
Low-Density Lipoprotein	136.04 +/- 4.23	123.92 +/- 4.17	122.84 +/- 4.17
Very Low-Density Lipoprotein	26.16 +/- 2.16	22.28 +/- 0.96	23.36 +/- 1.14

Mice aged 45–50 weeks were fed orally a dose of 600 mg/kg/head of cactus extracts once a day for 10 days. Control mice were treated only with 1ml of PBS without extract for 10 days. Source: "Effects of Cactus and Ginger Extracts as Dietary Antioxidants on Reactive Oxidant and Plasma Lipid Level," Food Science & Biotechnology, vol. 9, no. 2 (2000): pp. 83–99.

Discussion

The authors of the study acknowledge the generally known principle that LDL oxidized and accumulated by reactive oxidants narrows the artery and promotes atherosclerosis.[12] Therefore, they expect that dietary supplements of cactus and ginger extracts can reduce the oxidation of LDL and influence cholesterol levels in plasma. However, the scientists cannot explain a responsible mechanism at the time of the study. Nevertheless, they suggest that the reduction in plasma concentration of cholesterol comes from either reducing the different transformation of cholesterol content and preventing LDL from oxidizing by reactive oxidants or increasing the catabolic level of cholesterol by dietary antioxidants.

In conclusion, the authors suggest that the results of their analysis show that supplementation of cactus extracts can play a role as natural antioxidants. Further, these same extracts have a beneficial effect on blood lipids directly or indirectly in vivo.

TOXICITY

The prickly pear fruit is not toxic. No studies have reported acute or chronic toxicity reactions due to consumption of the cactus fruit or its products, of any species. Eating large quantities of the fresh fruit (30 to 50 fruits per day) might cause constipation due to the prevalence of the seeds. But not all people concur with this temporary side effect.

SUMMARY

Prickly pear pectin has been tested in humans and has been demonstrated to improve glucose response and plasma lipids in nondiabetic patients.[13] As determined in one of the earlier studies, individuals had significant decreases in plasma cholesterol and glucose after eight weeks of consumption of 9 g per day of pectin compared to the placebo group.[14] As shown in animal studies not included in this chapter, the oral intake of prickly pear pectin has exhibited a direct effect in reducing arteriosclerosis.[15] Clinical studies also showed that oral intake of pectin successfully reduced plasma LDL concentrations without having an effect on plasma HDL cholesterol or triglyceride concentrations.[16,17,18,19]

There is some question about the mechanism of action behind the fruit's medicinal effects. However, despite controversy over how the pectin operates within the body, the net result is always the same: a decrease in hepatic cholesterol concentrations in the user.

In conclusion, the intake of this soluble fiber appears to be beneficial for overall health. Prickly pear pectin has demonstrated some remarkable pharmacological effects in experimental studies. Its favorable effects are worth watching, as it may help reduce the incidence of some of the degenerative diseases of our time, including diabetes and coronary heart disease.[20] At the very minimum, the prickly pear fruit can be consumed as a preventive measure and as antioxidant support.

Other Benefits of and Treatments Using Prickly Pear Cactus

*Even since the time of the Aztecs, before the Spanish
people came to conquer Mexico, they said prickly pear
was good for any kind of disease.*
—Dr. Maria L. Fernandez[1]

The prickly pear cactus has a long tradition of use in other applications besides its utilization in the treatment and management of diabetes and cholesterol. This chapter contains information on peripheral ailments that the prickly pear cactus has been purported to heal. The information here has largely been derived from ethnobotanical sources based on the plant's long history of use. It should be noted that most of the time-honored medicinal claims in this chapter have not been substantiated by clinical research. This should not detract from the cactus's potential use in the treatment of the following self-limiting acute ailments. However, the cactus should not be substituted for medicine in the treatment of chronic ailments without further clinical evidence to fully support its use.

What follows is a compilation of primary uses of opuntia from generations of community medicinal use. Some of the claims are purely anecdotal, learned through experimentation and avid use, and they have been included in the research to present to you an objective understanding of the thoughts and practices surrounding the use of the herb by various global communities.

A LOT LIKE ALOE VERA

Little do most people know that the prickly pear and aloe vera have a lot in common. As a topical application, the pads of the prickly pear cactus, like aloe vera, appear to be first rate. Filleted prickly pear pads are thought to be excellent and very effective drawing poultices. Similar to aloe vera's application, they may be placed against the injured area, covered in gauze, and taped to the skin. After several hours, they are removed.

In 1989, Michael Moore, herb researcher and writer, wrote a very brief and concise description of nopal's use as a poultice and its mechanism of action. In his report he also compares the prickly pear to the aloe vera plant:

> Contusions, bruises and burns that are engorged and tender contain much feral blood and disorganized interstitial fluid. The mucopolysaccharide gel in the prickly pear flesh is strongly hydrophilic and hypertonic; some of the fluid exudates that build up in the injury are absorbed osmotically through the skin and into the cactus, while the gel softens the skin, decreases the tension against the injury, and lessens the pain. This is, by the way, how aloe vera works.[2]

For the purpose of this book, I would like to emphasize the similarity in both plants' use as a topical application. Examinations of their ethnobotany and history show that the preparations from the two succulents appear to be substitutable for similar models of inflammation and wound healing. Of course, additional research is required before such widespread use can be justified. However, the external application of the prickly pear cactus for its health-promoting effects is already a popular practice worldwide, as you will see in the ethnobotanical evidence presented in this chapter.

MORE USES OF CACTUS MEDICINE

Nopalea cochinillifera

Distribution: Can be found in southern Mexico, Guatemala, tropical America, the West Indies, and the Bahamas. Formerly grown commercially in the Americas and in the Canary Islands.

Medicinal Uses: In Mexico, joints are split open and the mucilaginous flesh is used as a poultice. There this cactus has a long record of use as a poultice on toothaches, earaches, rheumatic places, erysipelas, and inflamed eyes. The cooked joint is poulticed on abscesses. In Trinidad and elsewhere, it is often used as an emollient on burns and inflamed places. In the Yucatán an infusion of the flesh is used as a shampoo to stimulate hair growth. It is rubbed on the scalp daily. When the flesh of the cactus is applied to the abdomen and over the liver area, it helps to reduce internal inflammation and halt diarrhea.

When taken internally, it is reported to act as a diuretic in cases of urethritis, cystitis, and kidney complaints. In the Yucatán, a decoction of 35 g cubed joint is added to 1 pint of water and drunk 3 or 4 times per day, as is the customary dose. In Brazil, the fruit decoction is also taken to allay stomach or liver distress.[3]

Opuntia elatior

Distribution: This species of prickly pear is native to the Pacific coast of Costa Rica and Panama. It is also present in northern Colombia, Venezuela, Aruba, Bonaire, and Curaçao.

Medicinal Uses: The peeled joint is bound under the soles of the feet to draw out fever. [4]

Opuntia ficus-indica

Distribution: The cactus is common in the arid regions of Venezuela. It is cultivated in Bermuda, Cuba, Puerto Rico, the Virgin Islands, and Costa Rica. It is commercially grown throughout Mexico, the southwestern United States, Italy, and Israel for its fruits, pads, and flowers. This prickly pear was introduced and naturalized in the Mediterranean region of Europe and in Ethiopia and southern Africa.

Medicinal Uses: Before utilization of the pads, it is first recommended that they be roasted and crushed. This is a common practice among many users of different species of prickly pear all over the world. It is thought that warming the joints activates specific plant constituents.

A poultice of the cactus is applied on the liver area in cases of liver trouble. In Curaçao, the joints are peeled and warmed, then placed on the body to "draw out pain" (supposed analgesic properties). Because of its slightly astringent effect, an overnight infusion of the raw, chopped joints is taken internally to halt diarrhea and dysentery. It is also considered of special value for aiding the digestive process. This infusion is also drunk as a remedy for rabies.

A decoction of the peeled, cubed joint is drunk to relieve mild stomachache. It is used, too, as an enema in intestinal difficulties. Sweetened, it is frequently drunk to overcome chest complaints and high fevers. Also, it was formerly a treatment for gonorrhea. This same infusion can be applied externally on pimples and various skin diseases and for eye inflammation. In arid regions, the fresh pulp of the fruit is eaten to allay thirst. In Curaçao and Puerto Rico, the pulp is used for shampooing the hair.[5]

A small amount of research on the fruits of this species has shown it to have wound-healing and anti-inflammatory properties.[6,7] Most recently, the prickly pear was dubbed "The Workout Herb" in an article published by *Prevention* magazine in April 2003. A French research scientist, Gilles Gutierrez, established that professional athletes can work out longer and harder while using his patented cactus extract. Further, the herb sped their recoveries from strenuous exercise. Apparently, the cactus accelerates the body's natural restorative compounds.[8]

In addition to *Opuntia ficus-indica*'s uses as a wound healer, I have included below the summaries of two cactus flower clinical studies that have spawned discussion of the prickly pear's potential use in the treatment of benign prostatic hypertrophy (BPH). Though little research has been performed in this area, cactus flowers are already selling in the herbal market purportedly to treat symptoms of BPH.

Treatment of Benign Prostatic Hypertrophy with *Opuntia ficus-indica* (L.) Miller (*Journal of Herbs, Spices, & Medicinal Plants*)

Introduction

The objective of these clinical studies was to conduct a preliminary evaluation of the potential clinical application of opuntia flowers in the treatment of benign prostatic hypertrophy (BPH).[9] The authors acknowledge that several herbal folk medicine remedies and modern herbological preparations are currently used to ease BPH symptomology. Of these remedies, the most widely used are fruit from saw palmetto *(Serenoa repens)*, seeds from pumpkin *(Cucurbita pepo)*, vegetative tissue from horsetail *(Equisetum arvense)*, and roots and fruit from parsley *(Petroselinum crispum)*.

The prickly pear flowers also enjoy a reputation as a

remedy for urinary problems. In Sicily, a decoction made from the flower of this cactus is widely used as a strong diuretic.[10] In North Africa, the flowers are combined with barley seeds and corn silk to treat urinary obstruction.[11] The flowers of opuntia are included in the British Herbal Pharmacopoeia as a medicine with astringent and antihemorrhagic effects and can be used for colitis, diarrhea, and prostatic hypertrophy.[12] Incidentally, flowers from the cholla cactus are supposed to be interchangeable with prickly pear flowers.[13] Both flowers hail from the *Opuntia* cactus family.

Materials and Methods

Dried flowers of *Opuntia ficus-indica* (OFI) were collected in Israel. The collected flowers were sun-dried, ground to a powder, and packed into hard gelatin capsules for use in treatment of patients. Each capsule contained 250 mg of dried flower.

Two separate clinical trials were set up. The first was conducted at a private clinic and involved 58 male patients afflicted with BPH. Each patient was orally administered two gelatin capsules containing the dried, ground opuntia flowers three times per day. No control group was set up due to the preliminary nature of this study. The evaluation lasted six to eight months, and patients were questioned at the end of the trial with a set of subjective questions regarding symptoms of BPH.

The second trial was conducted at a urology outpatient clinic. It involved 30 BPH patients. The administration of opuntia was the same as in the first trial. This evaluation lasted two months instead of six months, however. Patients were questioned at both the beginning and end of the trial with the same list of questions. In addition, the subject underwent a physical examination before and after the trial. Urine was checked for blood, and the diameter of the urinary tract was measured by ultrasound. Urodynamic and microbiological tests were also used with the outpatient clinic patients to evaluate urinary tract function.

Results

In both trials, patients reported improvement in the symptoms of BPH following treatment. A large number of patients reported a decrease in the urgency to urinate, emergency urination, and a feeling of fullness in the bladder. Not all patients received relief from symptoms following treatment, however. In addition, the response to different symptoms was mixed. The investigators noted no toxicity and no deterioration in urinary function. See table 6.1 for full results of the two clinical studies.

Limitations

The results of this study are encouraging; however, there are several limitations to the study that should be addressed, including the following:

- The two studies were conducted for different time spans, making the results difficult to compare.
- There is no explanation for the percentage of disparity that exists between both sets of patient in terms of improvement: specifically, in urgency of urination and drops after voiding.

TABLE 6.1
EVALUATION OF CACTUS FLOWERS IN TREATMENT OF BPH

Urinary Complaint	CLINICAL TRIAL		
	PRIVATE	UROLOGY OUTPATIENT	
	(% improved)	(% complaints)	(% improved)
Urgency for urination	50.0%	92.5%	80.0%
Emergency urination	62.0%	85.2%	52.2%
Feeling of bladder fullness	46.0%	92.5%	48.0%
Drops after voiding	63.0%	66.7%	33.3%
Nocturia (>2x/night)	------*	100.0%	33.3%

Source: Journal of Herbs, Spices & Medicinal Plants, *vol. 2 (1) 1993.*
*Not recorded in private study.

- Nocturia was not recorded in the private clinical study, so it is difficult to evaluate its improvement against the outpatient test group.
- The dose-response relationship needs to be further explored. What are the optimal doses? Might a larger dose with greater frequency affect the user and improve symptomology? Also, why did patients at the private clinic cite less improvement for urgency of urination than the group of outpatients, given six additional months of treatment?

These criticisms of the study are tempered by the fact that this study was only intended to be a preliminary evaluation of the clinical application of cactus flowers. The physicians who conducted these trials were aware of its limitations. At the time of this study, a double-blind crossover, placebo-controlled trial with 100 patients, lasting eight to twelve months, was in progress.

Cactus Flower Extracts May Prove Beneficial in Benign Prostatic Hyperplasia due to Inhibitor of 5-alpha Activity, Aromatase Activity and Lipid Peroxidation *(Urological Research)*

The cactus flower is deemed helpful in benign prostate hyperplasia (BPH) therapy (British Herbal Pharmacopoeia, 1983), although there is no published information regarding its clinical effects on patients or the mechanism of its biological activity. The purpose of this study was to evaluate the 5-alpha reductase inhibition, aromatase inhibition, and antioxidant potential of cactus flower extract known as opuntia.[14] Researchers found the cactus extract had ameliorative effects on prostate hyperplasia. This action was attributable to numerous as yet unidentified compounds that inhibited prostatic 5-alpha reductase and aromatase acivity. The researchers were positive on their initial results and recognize that additional clinical trials are required to examine and verify the full significance of cactus flower extracts in the treatment of BPH.

Opuntia sillenii and *Opuntia dillenii* (Haw.)

Distribution: This species can be found growing in the most diametrically opposed conditions. It is common from Texas to Florida, and is also found in Bermuda, throughout the Bahamas, the West Indies, and from southeastern Mexico to northern South America, Africa, Pakistan, India, and Australia.

Medicinal Uses: In the Bahamas, the mucilaginous flesh of the joints is beaten in water and drunk to relieve urinary burning. This same decoction when mixed with various local herbs is taken as a remedy for tuberculosis. It is poulticed on boils and cuts, and on the foot as a cold remedy. As a treatment for stomach ulcers, the flesh of 3 joints are boiled in 1 l of water for 1 to 2 hours, then drunk as needed.

In Haiti, the joint is roasted and ground, then applied on tumors. In the Yucatán, the joints are heated and applied as poultices to relieve pleurisy. The Bahamians report that the cactus has the effect of minimizing arthritic and rheumatic pains when applied as a poultice. Since medicated shampoos are either not available or too expensive, the crushed joints of the prickly pear can be utilized as a shampoo to combat dandruff.[15]

Opuntia streptacantha

Distribution: Very common on the Mexican tablelands.

Medicinal Uses: Like other species of prickly pear cacti, it has similar topical applications. A recent clinical study conducted in the United Kingdom and later published in the journal *Antiviral Research* demonstrated the antiviral properties of the OS extract.[16] It is well known that certain plant extracts will inhibit virus replication and will inactivate extracellular viruses. The purpose of this initial study was to examine inhibition of replication of DNA and RNA viruses by extracts of OS, the nature of the active components, and preliminary evidence of safety in human and nonhuman species.

An extract of the cactus plant was found effective in inhibiting intracellular virus replication and inactivating extracellular virus. Inhibition of virus replication also occurred following pre-infection treatment—a favorable finding in terms of in vivo limitation of virus disease. There was inhibition of both DNA and RNA virus replication, for example, herpes simplex virus, equine herpes virus, psuedorabies virus, influenza virus, respiratory syncytial virus, and human immunodeficiency virus, with normal protein synthesis in uninfected cells.

The active inhibitory component(s) appeared to be protein in nature and resided in the wall of the plant rather than in the cuticle or inner sap. This is valuable to know, as the pads should not be peeled before use. The mechanism of action of the active components of the extract is presently unknown. The scientists suggest, however, that the active component might be protein, thus making it distinct from the alkaloid-flavonoid group of viral inhibitors.

The extract was nontoxic on oral administration to humans, mice, and horses. Human patients received 3 g/day for 6 months. There were no adverse reactions by oral administration. This herb shows much promise for the treatment of viruses. The results of this study were very encouraging and point to a new, open door in the wide range of prickly pear pharmacological activity.

Opuntia Wentiana

Distribution: This species is native and extremely abundant on the islands of Aruba, Bonaire, and Curaçao. It also grows in Colombia and Venezuela, up to 55 meters above sea level.

Medicinal Uses: Like so many of the uses above, the peeled joints are applied as emollient poultices to cuts, sores, and burns. A root decoction is drunk 3 times per day and is considered to be a remedy in relief of asthma and kidney pain. Again, we see that a hot-water infusion of the flesh of a joint is good for any stomach disorder. The joints are also said to be good for swollen feet. To reduce swelling of feet in fishermen, and others after prolonged sitting, a cloth is soaked in the cool root decoction and applied to the swollen area.[17]

FURTHER USES OF THE PADS AND FRUITS

The following material is taken from Daniel E. Moerman's "Medicinal Plants of Native America, Research Reports in Ethnobotany."[18]

Analgesic: The Shoshone applied a poultice from the inner pulp of the fruit to cuts and wounds for faster healing and reduction of pain. *(Opuntia basilaris)*

Anti-inflammatory diuretic: When there is pain on urination, with a continuing dull ache in the urethra and bladder well after completion, the juice can be taken to decrease pain. In Mexico, a teaspoon is recommended every two hours until the pain is gone. This is only taken to relieve the inflammation; it does not affect any of the bacteria that may be causing the pain.

Antirheumatic: The Costanoan applied a poultice of warm fruit on rheumatism. Warm fruit juice was also rubbed on the affected area. *(Opuntia streptacantha)*

Astringent: Eating the fruit has been recommended for diarrhea, due to its high pectin content.

Bone healer: Still today, the flesh of the prickly pear is used to mend broken bones. The pads are toasted, sliced in half, and then each half is placed on either side of the fracture.

Hemostat: The peeled joints were used by the Kiowa as an instrument for compressing a blood vessel. *(Opuntia streptacantha)*

Male aphrodisiac: A leading manufacturer of prickly pear foods in the United States sells the fruits to the Korean pharmaceutical market for its supposed prostate-healing and aphrodisiac properties.

Poison: The species of prickly pear was used by the Navajo as a poison for hunting. *(Opuntia polyacantha)*

Throat aid: The Shuswap applied a poultice to a swollen throat. *(Opuntia fragilis)*

Water purifier: Drop a filleted pad in the water. Spoon the grime that will rise up to the surface of the water.

Dermatological Aid

Various Native American tribes have used different species of the prickly pear cactus as a dermatological aid.[19]

- Dakota: A poultice of peeled stems was bound on wounds. *(Opuntia humifusa)*
- Kiowa: Thorns used to puncture the skin of boils. *(Opuntia streptacantha)*
- Mahuna: Flowers of the fruit were inserted into wounds. *(Opuntia streptacantha)*
- Nanticoke: The juice of the fruit was rubbed on warts. *(Opuntia humifusa)*
- Navajo: The spines were formerly used to pierce ears and lance small skin abscesses. *(Opuntia plumbea)*
- Pawnee: A poultice of peeled stems was bound on wounds. *(Opuntia humifusa)*
- Shoshone: Glochids were rubbed into warts or moles to remove them. *(Opuntia basilaris)*
- Shuswap: A poultice of heated quills was applied to cuts, sores, or boils. *(Opuntia fragilis)*

Gynecological Aid

Various Native American tribes have used different species of the prickly pear cactus as a gynecological aid.[20]

- Lummi: The mother-to-be drank an infusion of smashed pads in order to facilitate childbirth. *(Opuntia streptacantha)*
- Navajo: Peeled joints were roasted and the mucilage was used to lubricate the midwife's hand for placenta removal. *(Opuntia plumbea)*
- Pima: The poultice of a heated plant was applied to the breasts to encourage the flow of milk. *(Opuntia engelmannii* and *Opuntia phaeacantha)*

Application and Dosage
of Prickly Pear Cactus

O true apothecary! Thy drugs are quick.
—William Shakespeare, *Romeo and Juliet*

As no detailed clinical studies have determined which specific commercially prepared prickly pear products should be used for preventive measures and which should be used in the treatment of disease, the following is offered only as a dosage guideline based on the studies included in this book and their historical use. The type of preparation, source material, and the user's intention are all cofactors in choosing the proper dosage. Further, the quality of the source material hinges on the level of certain constituents found in the medicine per soil quality, species, and maturity when harvested.

BLOOD SUGAR MANAGEMENT
(Prickly Pear Pads)

You are most likely to see pads from the *Opuntia streptacantha* or *Opuntia ficus-indica* variety used in the treatment of diabetes or management of blood sugar levels. It is believed that heating the extracts or the entire stems prior to administration might be necessary in order to elicit the antidiabetic effect. However, several successful test studies have documented the effectiveness of utilizing fresh raw pads. The doses and uses listed in this section may also be used for health maintenance.

Bulk: The cactus was usually administered in one of two ways. Either 4 oz of fresh-pressed juice was drunk per day, or 500 g of broiled nopal stems were consumed daily. If you choose you may increase this dosage, as no side effects or toxicity have been reported from increased consumption.

Capsules: If you choose to administer encapsulated nopal, follow the directions on the label and/or separate company instructions, as there is no standard dosage available because capsule size varies. Dosage might also vary given the species of nopal. The average dose is 2 capsules (325–650 milligrams), three times per day.

Infusions: The cactus pads can be safely ingested in liquid form. When the cactus is taken as an infusion, the average suggested dosage is 1 tablespoon three to four times per day. Dosage varies according to ailment and can be increased or decreased as needed. Use the following example as a guideline: in the treatment of an acute disorder, such as cystitis, a tablespoon may be administered every two hours until the pain is gone.

Tinctures: The juice of the fresh plant can be preserved by alcohol. However, too much use of the extract, equal to the portions of the fresh plant, would supply enough alcohol to create a blood sugar problem. It is advised that you purchase tinctures that utilize stabilizers other than alcohol.

Fruit syrup or nectar: Follow the directions on the label, as dosage may vary per fruit concentration. Be sure to check for the presence of refined sugar.

CHOLESTEROL MANAGEMENT
(Prickly Pear Fruits)

A daily dose of 5 to 9 grams per day of prickly pear fruit pectin may be effective in the prevention or reversal of a hypocholesterolemic condition, though some studies showed that lower doses of 2.50 g of prickly pear pectin demonstrated effectiveness.

Bulk: The average-sized fruit contains approximately 3.60 g of dietary fiber. Eating 3 fruits per day would double the minimum treatment requirement. This dosage would then not only help to satisfy daily vitamin and mineral nutritional requirements, but would also serve up a healthy dose of flavonoids.

Syrups or nectars: Dosage will vary. While some companies might choose to utilize sugar in the formula, others might substitute sugar with other natural sweeteners.

Jellies, jams, marmalades, and candy: If you choose to get your pectin content from foods be sure to examine which particular species of opuntia has been used in the preparation of the product. Recognize that commercially prepared cactus foods are not a substitute for any traditional forms of medication or for specially prepared fruit nectars.

Juice: The juice tastes great, but will not supply you with pectin, the key ingredient responsible for the lowering of plasma cholesterol levels. You will, however, receive a nutritional shot of vitamins, minerals, and flavonoids.

GENERAL IMMUNE SYSTEM BUILDER
(Prickly Pear Flowers)

It is now estimated that the average daily intake of total flavonoids in the United States is about 25 milligrams. An intake greater than 30 milligrams significantly reduces the risk of cardiovascular mortality.[1]

Bulk: One small dried flower in a well-strained infusion. One cup, three times a day. For larger flowers, a few petals per cup of hot water, three times a day.

Capsules: 325 to 650 mg, three times per day. Or place two capsules in one cup of hot water as an infusion.

Tincture (1:5): 3 to 4 ml, three times daily.

Infusion: Add two tea bags to a pot of hot water. Drink one cup three times a day.

QUESTIONS AND ANSWERS

Q. Can I self-medicate with the prickly pear cactus?

A. The Food and Drug Administration (FDA) mandates over-the-counter (OTC) drugs to treat self-limiting, acute ailments. It's best that you utilize the prickly pear cactus as you would an OTC product. It is permissible to administer the cactus as a general immune system builder. However, if you wish to utilize the cactus in the treatment of diabetes or high plasma cholesterol levels, then professional medical supervision is recommended.

Q. Should I stop taking my diabetes medication when I first try the nopal?

A. If you are under doctor supervision and have been advised by your doctor to quit your prescription medication, then I advise you to follow your doctor's orders. It is best not to substitute any medications without professional supervision. Talk to your doctor about your options.

Q. Should I stop taking my cholesterol medication when I first try the pads or the cactus pears?

A. The answer to this question is the same as the previous answer. It would be dangerous to quit any medication without medical supervision. Cholesterol levels need to be monitored frequently. Oral consumption of the prickly pear pads or fruits is not a substitute for medical care. Self-medication for chronic ailments is not advised.

Q. Will I get the same results as those from the clinical studies?

A. Nobody can give you absolute assurance that the prickly pear cactus will positively affect you. Not even a prescription drug maker can offer you this level of assurance of their drugs. Treating a person is as much of an art as it is a science. Doctors are aware that a person may display a different reaction to any foreign substance. Nevertheless, given the integrity of the prickly pear clinical trials, and the use of a high-quality prickly pear, it's very possible that you will experience positive benefits.

Q. Is the prickly pear cactus addictive? Will I be able to stop once I have started?

A. None of the clinical research conducted to date has shown that the prickly pear cactus is addictive. It has a long history of use all over the world as a food with no reported addictions.

Q. How can I be sure of the quality of the prickly pear cactus medicine that I purchase (e.g., teas, capsules, and syrups)?

A. The natural products industry is a self-regulated industry at this time, though they conform to the rules set forth by the

FDA. Some companies elect to be members of an industry trade association such as the NNFA (National Nutrition Foods Association) to have their products third-party tested and approved. For the most part, quality and integrity of product is left to market forces to decide. Be sure to buy only those products that are manufactured by companies of integrity and good standing in the natural foods marketplace, public or private.

Q. What if I can't find any prickly pear products at my local grocery store or natural products food store?

A. Refer to the resource section at the back of this book for a list of companies that sell the prickly pear cactus as food and medicine. Some of them are capable of online order fulfillment.

Q. What if I am only interested in eating the prickly pear cactus as a food, but not taking it as a medicine?

A. Before the cactus was recognized as a medicine, it was a food. Eat it whenever you feel like it and don't pay any attention to the guidelines of dosage included in this chapter. As the prickly pear cactus is a nutritive food, you can certainly expect to indirectly receive some health benefits.

Q. Can I take all three parts of the cactus at the same time? For example, may I consume the prickly pear pad capsules while I drink the tea and later eat the fruit?

A. Absolutely. There are no contraindications to mixing the three components. As they taste different, your taste buds won't even realize that they all came from the same source.

Q. I would like to drink the cactus flower infusion, but can I add something to jazz it up while not mitigating its health benefits?

A. Yes. One manufacturer I know combines its cactus petals with lemon peel to give additional flavor and provide an additional flavonoid boost. You can also add some stevia, a natural sweetener, to the infusion if you want sweetness and are concerned about blood sugar levels. Cactus flowers also make for a great iced tea.

Picking and Preparing the Prickly Pear

Spines and serpents aside, the prickly pear is a highly accessible cactus. It seems to grow most everywhere . . . it [is] supply waiting for demand.
—Arizona Highways[1]

Whether you are interested in escaping to the wild to find your own cactus or going to the supermarket to pick it off the shelves, this chapter is for you. It is divided into three sections: "Prickly Pear Pads," "Prickly Pear Fruits," and "Prickly Pear Flowers." In each section, I write about how to properly identify, collect, and prepare the different parts of the prickly pear cactus.

The great thing about collecting the prickly pear is that it is easy, inexpensive, and fun. However, if you aren't interested in doing any of the work yourself and you would rather buy the commercially prepared cactus products, then you can skip to the "At the Supermarket" and "At the Health Food Store" headings in each of the three sections. There you will find the information that you need to choose from the many varieties of prickly pear products that you will find on the grocery and natural food store shelves.

PRICKLY PEAR PADS

Identifying the Right Pads

Whether you are going to be picking pads for use as medicine or food, you are going to need to know how to choose the best pads available. The questions you should be asking yourself include: When can I pick the best pads? What pads look the healthiest? Which ones will taste best?

The healthiest looking pads always make for the most therapeutically active medicines, so be sure to look for thick, swollen joints. When the joints are swollen it means they are engorged with water and gel. They should be thick, soft to the touch, and slightly flexible when bent. You will easily be able to distinguish between a swollen pad and one that is dried up. It is the difference between a football and a Frisbee. Choosing a dried-up, thin pad will probably not exhibit much of a medicinal effect due to its lesser water and gel content.

When the pads are to be prepared as medicine, they can be picked at any time of the year because their medicinal activity is not influenced by season. If, however, you are only locating thin, dried-up pads, and are having difficulty finding freshly swollen joints, you may want to search for pads after a period of rainfall. This way the pads have time to absorb and store their water.

When the pads are going to be specifically prepared as food, the younger, small dark green, tender pads should be chosen. Most cultures that prepare the nopal as a vegetable in meals prefer the young pads. These too should be swollen and slightly flexible when bent. The younger pads are more abundant in spring or after a period of rainfall. Once picked, the pads will stay fresh for up to two weeks if stored in an airtight container in the refrigerator.

Collecting the Wild Pads

To harvest the fresh pads, remove them with tongs at the point where they join the old tough pads. When choosing between different species of prickly pear, you will see that some cacti have spines while others do not. The presence of spines should not influence your choice of pads. No matter how many spines are on an individual pad, you should be able to remove them without any problem. Just make certain to always look for the healthiest-looking cactus.

A Word of Caution on Collecting Wild Pads

There are many species of the prickly pear cactus growing around the world. One should always exercise caution when ingesting any unrecognized wild prickly pear. Certain species of nopal are poisonous and are not safe for consumption. Fortunately, the poisonous nopal are very few and far between, so the chances of you stumbling upon one are rare. But do not test your luck. Unless you have someone knowledgeable accompanying you on your herb search it is best to not ingest any wild plants.

In some states, including Arizona, it is against the law to pick the pads of the prickly pear growing in the wild. So check with the Fish and Game Department in your state to learn what the laws are in your area. No one wants to have to pay a fine for picking a pad. Harvesting the pads on private property is okay as long as you have permission.

Preparing the Fresh Pads

Let's say that by now you have collected your first set of prickly pear pads, and are sitting in the kitchen wondering how on earth you are going to cook these green things (sometimes the pads are purple so they would be called "purple things"; you get the idea).

To prepare the pads for cooking, the first step is to parboil them for 10 to 20 minutes until firm yet tender. If you wish, you may add a large clove of garlic or a slice of onion to the water for flavor. The Hopi Indians, for instance, added an ear of sweet corn for flavoring. After the allotted time, drain.

Next, the pads must be cleaned. The easiest way to clean a pad is to grasp it in one hand, place it on a cutting board, and with a paring knife scrape off the spines and eyes. If you do not have a paring knife, an ordinary kitchen peeler will do. Perform this activity under cold running water, then rinse thoroughly and inspect for stickers. Since there are usually many thorns on either side of a pad, it is best to trim away about one-sixteenth of the edge. Also, trim portions of the pad wherever it is bruised, dry, or tough. Next, wash again. With the end of a potato peeler, you can cut around the spiny nodules to remove them.

Some like to parboil the pads an additional one or two times, followed by a rinsing of the pads in cold water. However many times you choose to parboil the pads is a matter of your personal preparation style. Some prefer additional parboiling since the process lowers the pad's oxalic acid content. If you eat nopal every day and are concerned with your calcium level, you may want to follow this method, as daily intake of oxalic acid in large doses may interfere with calcium absorption. However, additional parboiling also removes some of the mucilage content. Infrequent users need only parboil one time.

Once the pads are clean of grime and thorns, scrutinize each pad carefully under sufficient lighting in order to see whether or not all the thorns have been removed. It is better to get a thorn in your finger now than in your tongue or lip later. If there are no thorns on the pad, it is ready for cooking. Remember to clean your knife and cutting board before you "de-sticker" other pads to prevent new pads from getting stuck with stray thorns.

Juicing the Pads

Some might prefer to juice the raw or cooked pads rather than to consume them as a meal. If you want to juice the pads you can chop up the skinned inner flesh and then puree the cactus in a blender. The contents in the blender are referred to as prickly pear slurry. This method is easy, does not take much time, and you can drink it as is. Other vegetables, herbs, or sweeteners can be added for flavor or for an added punch of nutritive value.

Teas, Infusions, and Decoctions

The most common method of preparing herbs for oral consumption is to make a tea. This involves adding hot water to dried plant material—such as bark, berries, flowers, leaves, roots, or seeds. The hot water serves as a solvent in extracting some of the plant material's biologically active components. Some herbs lend themselves well to this process, particularly plants with aerial, or aboveground, parts.[2]

An infusion is basically the same as tea. After the herbal tea bag steeps in hot water for a period of time, a process called *infusing*, it becomes a type of herbal extract known as an *infusion*.

Roots, barks, seeds, and berries tend to require a little more heat and time to release their medicinal compounds. These usually need to be simmered over low heat for anywhere from 10 to 30 minutes. Herbal practitioners refer to this process as *decocting* and the product it yields as a *decoction*.

If you choose to follow some of the practices of various cultures in the administration of the prickly pear, you may either prepare an infusion or decoction. Both methods of preparation are very similar but the latter will require additional time for steeping.

At the Supermarket

If you find these directions too time-consuming or tedious, you can always opt to buy canned or jarred prickly pear pads at the supermarket. Though they are not fresh, they still taste good. They are generally found in the Mexican food section of the store.

If prepackaged cactus does not suit your taste, fresh pads should be available in the produce department of your grocery store. In some places, you might have to go to the "exotic" produce section to locate the pads. In Arizona, it is always funny to find the pads sitting in the exotic food section of any grocery store since the cactus is, more than likely, growing right near the supermarket's front parking lot.

If your store does not carry them, speak to the manager about purchasing the prickly pear. If the state of Texas can import forty thousand pounds of prickly pear pads a day from Mexico, then your supermarket should not have a problem with receiving a limited supply. Pick the medium-sized, firm pads and avoid purchasing limp, dry, or soggy pads.

At the Health Food Store

Your natural foods store should stock the canned, jarred, or fresh pads. In addition to these, they are most likely to carry other commercially prepared varieties of the pads, including the dried encapsulated pads, powdered nopal, extracts, and tinctures. The cactus pads will usually be bottled under the name of cactus, nopal, or opuntia. Most companies sell either the *Opuntia streptacantha* or *Opuntia ficus-indica* variety.

The prickly pear pads are also included in a number of different combination items geared toward various applications such as diabetes, cholesterol management, or wound healing. Multiherb commercial preparations offer several advantages, such as the encapsulation of similarly acting herbs to optimize each plant's medicinal effectiveness.

PRICKLY PEAR FRUITS

Identifying the Cactus Fruits

When picking cactus fruit for the first time, there are a few things to know. First, August to mid-September offer the best opportunities to pick cactus fruit. During this period, the fruit is most ripe. Second, the fruits are easy to spot since they grow directly from the pads. The skin of the fruit is dry and tough to the touch. The tasty, fleshy inner part is much softer and contains about 85 percent water.

There will be different-colored fruit available depending on the environment the cactus grows in and the particular species of cactus you pick from. Colors of the fruit range from dull red to reddish-purple, and bright yellow to green, and even include marmalade orange. The flavor of all varieties tastes somewhat the same. The level of sweetness and pectin concentration depends on factors such as the species of fruit, soil quality, rainfall, temperature, elevation, and fruit maturity. The fruits, of course, taste best when they are ripe.

But how can you tell when a cactus fruit is ready to be picked and eaten? There are several ways you can recognize fruit maturity. First, you can perform a cursory examination of the skin of the fruit while it is still attached to the pad.

Second, you can lightly twist the fruit. If it rips easily from the cactus, the fruit is most likely ready for eating. If the fruit doesn't budge, then it has not yet reached its full stage of maturity. It needs more time to grow to create its sweet and juicy flavor.

Collecting the Cactus Fruits

The skin of the fruit lacks spines, but does have many glochids. These glochids are tiny thorns, barely visible to the eye. If you examine the fruit carefully, you will be able to see them. Through normal handling, these peach fuzz barbed wires can easily work their way into the flesh. They are not poisonous. Glochids are more annoying than dangerous or painful.

Tongs should be used to collect the tuna to avoid getting a number of glochids stuck in your skin. If you don't want to use tongs, then I strongly recommend you wear gloves when collecting the prickly pear fruits. Also, when picking your own fruits, resist tasting them immediately unless you are very careful of the thorns. There are no thorns on the inside of the fruit. But unknowingly, people who peel the fruit with their hands will probably transfer some of those stickers to their mouths. This can result in a disquieting afternoon with glochids in your lips and gums from unwise munching. If the stickers do penetrate your mouth, though they are impossible to see, they do dislodge or dissolve within seven or eight hours.

As far as the fruits are concerned, there is no law against harvesting them in any state. You can legally pick them from prickly pear cacti growing in the wild, though you might not be able to purloin their pads.

Preparing the Cactus Fruits

You can prepare the fruit one of two ways. The first involves grabbing a stiff brush and scrubbing the fruit under running water to remove some of the stickers. Then, with a knife, peel the skin from the fruit. Once peeled, the tuna is ready to be eaten or included in one of your recipes.

The other way of preparing the tuna is almost identical. First, brush the fruits under running water just as you did in the previous method. Next, place the pears in boiling water and blanch for about 10 seconds. Remove the pears from the water with tongs. Now, the fruits have been quickly heated so the thorns are less irritating, and peeling the fruit becomes easier. Blanch and cool only six at a time, because once the fruits cool the thorns become stiff again. The peels can be discarded.

Juicing the Cactus Fruits

There is no special formula for juicing the fruits: You only need to peel the skin, cut the fruit, and throw it into the blender. Make sure you do not mistakenly throw the peel into the blender, as it is not edible.

At the Supermarket

For people who elect not to bother with the gloves and blanching, the option to purchase the fresh fruit at the store is always open. The fresh fruits, like the pads, usually sit in the "exotic" section of the produce department. I have seen the pads readily available in grocery stores in larger cities across the United States.

The fruits are also sold in a number of different commercial preparations including nectars, jellies, jams, candies, barbecue sauces, salsas, and nectars. These foods are also commonly sold at gift shops in the Southwest.

At the Health Food Store

Your local health food store might stock both the fresh fruits and the commercially prepared foods made from the prickly pear cactus fruits. In addition, they might also sell no-sugar-added cactus fruit products, given that many of its users may be concerned with blood sugar levels. Other forms of administration include extracts, tinctures, and freeze-dried capsules. The fruits will generally be bottled under one of the following names: prickly pear fruit, cactus fruit, cactus pear, or Indian figs.

Mucho Seeds

The cactus pear contains a lot of seeds. These seeds are safe for consumption, though some Native American tribes claim that eating too many can cause stomach discomfort. I have eaten up to fifteen fruits in one sitting and have not once experienced any sort of discomfort.

During the harvest in Mexico in the early 1900s, whole families hiked up into the hills and camped out in "Nopaleros," practically living on tunas alone. It was not out of the ordinary for an individual to eat two hundred per day![3] It is difficult for me to imagine eating twenty tunas a day, much less two hundred.

PRICKLY PEAR FLOWERS

Identifying and Collecting the Cactus Flowers

Prickly Pear flowering usually starts in mid-May and lasts until mid-June, but fertilization and irrigation can also achieve autumn flowering. The flowers are easy to identify because they are shaped like roses and grow directly from the fruits.

Gathering the flowers is an easy task. But you may want to wear gloves when you harvest them because the flowers of most species are surrounded by glochids. Place the flowers in a bag while you are collecting. As a rule, the red-colored flowers contain the highest concentration of biologically active flavonoids.

No law exists that I am aware of that limits the harvesting of prickly pear flowers.

Preparing the Fresh Flowers

When you are finished picking the flowers, it is time for them to be dried. Place the flowers in a cardboard carton. The petals will dry best in shaded areas with adequate circulation. They should not be placed in direct sunlight. Once the botanicals are dry, they should be stored in glass jars and placed in a cool, dark area such as a cupboard or cabinet.

When you are ready to prepare the infusion, add one whole dried flower to one cup of hot water. For larger flowers, adding only one or two petals will be enough. Make sure that you strain the infusion well to prevent the swallowing of glochid hairs, which can irritate your throat but are not otherwise harmful.

At the Health Food Store

If picking the flowers and getting a glochid or two stuck in your palm is not for you, then you can buy the cactus flowers already prepared in tea bags at your local health food store. The store might also carry the flower petals in bulk, so be sure to check. Most likely, the tea bags will not be for sale at your local supermarket, though the store will probably carry some version of the pads or fruits.

Cactus Cooking

You don't have to cook fancy or complicated
masterpieces—just good food from fresh ingredients.
—Julia Child

THE FIRST TIME I ATE THE PRICKLY PEAR

The first time I tried the prickly pear was during a trip to Mexico several years ago. The excursion to Mexico was meant to be a short trip and its purpose was pure and simple R&R. I didn't go down there to search for any exotic herbs.

But one early Sunday morning after a Saturday night of lively dancing, I was invited to breakfast at a friend's house. Delia wanted to cook an authentic homemade Mexican breakfast for me. I accepted the invitation and caught a cab outside the hotel.

When I arrived at Delia's I was greeted by her daughter, Alma, and her husband, Gustavo, who stood at the countertop in the corner of the kitchen scrubbing long green vegetable pads. The pads measured approximately 3 to 4 inches wide and about $1/2$ to $3/4$ inches thick and were a dark iguana green color. He gently scrubbed the pads with a wire brush, diligently moving the brush in a vertical motion as if he was scraping a piece of burned toast. As he brushed the cactus pad, he managed to pull out several stickers, or thorns, as they are commonly called.

"What are you doing?" I inquired.

"Preparing the nopales," he answered. "The nopal has a very special flavor. It is *bueno* [good] for the stomach and for a long life. The Indians call nopal a longevity tonic. As you can see, Ran, the nopal has been very good to me. I still work, and I am seventy-one years old."

He finished cleaning the pads and then dumped them in a pot of boiling water. He allowed them to cook for six or seven minutes to make them soft.

That morning, the first time I ate prickly pear, Delia and Gustavo prepared nopal eggs for breakfast, a recipe provided later in this chapter. Cooked together with the egg and a little bit of pepper and cilantro, it's a healthy and tasty meal. The prickly pear joints make a delectable vegetable dish, with a taste similar to slightly peppery green beans and containing mucilage that is reminiscent of okra. Like any other vegetable, they can be sliced, cooked, and seasoned to suit any palate. Due to its versatility, the prickly pear can be prepared with virtually any dish, or eaten alone.

CACTUS IN THE KITCHEN

Some prickly pear recipes are finding their way into the vegetable and fruit sections of general cookbooks, but mostly these recipes are limited to cookbooks on Southwestern and Mexican cookery. The following recipes offer some of the tastiest prickly pear dishes, juices, jellies, and treats using both the pads and the fruits. There are both traditional and modern recipes that are all simple and easy to prepare. If you enjoy experimenting with new flavors, then you will certainly welcome the following food preparations. In fact, some of these recipes are so delicious that you may get permanently hooked on the cactus (no pun intended).[1]

COOKING WITH CACTUS PADS

Note: Tofu or tempeh products can be adequately substituted for meat in the following recipes.

SHISH-KEBAB

Marinade
$1/4$ clove garlic, minced
2 tablespoons minced onion
$1/8$ teaspoon oregano
$1/16$ teaspoon thyme
$1/8$ teaspoon pepper
$1/4$ teaspoon salt
2 tablespoon vegetable oil
4 teaspoon white vinegar

Skewer food
$1/2$ pound flank steak
8 cherry tomatoes
$1/2$ cup pineapple chunks
$1/2$ cup chopped pads, cut into chunks and parboiled
8 fresh mushrooms
8 small white onions, parboiled

Combine the ingredients of the marinade and add the meat chunks. Let the meat marinate in sauce overnight in the refrigerator. Next, place the vegetables on skewers, making sure to alternate them. Place them over hot coals or broil in the oven until the meat reaches the desired doneness. During cooking, baste the kebabs with the marinade. Serves 3–4.

BEAVER TAIL STEW

1 cup nopal
$1/4$ cup chopped onion
Safflower oil, for frying
1 teaspoon sea salt

2 cloves garlic, finely minced
1 large tomato or 2 small tomatoes, chopped
1 to 2 tablespoons chili paste
2 shakes cumin
$^1/_2$ cup cooked shredded pork, venison, or tofu

Fry the nopal and the onion in the oil until they are slightly crisp. Add the salt, garlic, tomato, chili paste, cumin, and tofu or meat. Simmer until the tomato is done. If the tomato was not very juicy, add water or tomato juice so the mixture can simmer without burning. Serve with tortillas. Serves 1–2.

GRILLED CACTUS PADS

You'll love eating this next time you have a cookout.

2 cactus pads
Olive oil, for basting

Grill the pads over a charcoal fire for 10 to 12 minutes on each side. Thicker leaves may take longer to grill. Brush the leaves occasionally with the olive oil. Serve hot. Serves 1–2.

PEPPER STEAK

$^1/_2$ pound flank steak (use meat tenderizer, if desired)
$^1/_2$ cup chopped onions
$^1/_4$ cup beef broth, or use bouillon
1 tablespoon soy sauce
$^1/_2$ clove garlic, minced
$^1/_2$ cup nopal strips
$1^1/_2$ teaspoons cornstarch
5 tablespoons cold water
4 cherry tomatoes, quartered

Brown the meat. Add the onions and cook until soft. Add the broth, soy sauce, nopal, and garlic. Cover and simmer for 10 minutes. Blend together the cornstarch and water, and add to the meat mixture. Cook until thickened. Add the tomatoes and cook until heated through. Serves 3–4.

THREE-VEGETABLE SALAD

Dressing
$1/2$ cup vinegar
$1/2$ cup vegetable oil of choice
$1/2$ cup raw sugar
1 teaspoon salt
$1/2$ teaspoon pepper

Salad
1 cup nopales, cut in $1/4$-by-1-inch strips and parboiled
1 cup red bell pepper, cut the same and parboiled
$1/2$ to $3/4$ cup onion rings, sliced very thin

Mix the dressing in a blender or mixer until the sugar is thoroughly dissolved. Add the dressing to the vegetables in a bowl, cover, and refrigerate. The salad will keep for several days. Serves 2.

NOPALES AND EGGS (NOPAL EGGS)

2 tablespoons finely chopped onion
1 tablespoon oil or butter
2 tablespoons diced nopal
4 eggs, beaten
1 tablespoon water
Sea salt and pepper

In a heavy pan over medium heat, sauté the onion in the oil or butter until transparent. Add the nopal and heat thoroughly. Beat the eggs and water. Reduce the heat to low, and after the frying pan has cooled slightly, add the eggs and scramble. Season with the salt and pepper to taste. Some persons may prefer to use high-oleic safflower oil instead of butter. Serves 2.

CACTUS CONDIMENT

1/4 cup chopped onion (Spanish or green or a combination)
Safflower oil, for frying
1/4 cup nopal
3 tablespoons red chili paste
1/2 cup water

Sauté the onion in the oil until transparent. Add the nopal and fry for about 1 minute. Add the red chili paste and water. Simmer until the pads are well saturated with sauce. Use as a sauce for a meat or tofu dish. Serves 1–2.

COOKING WITH CACTUS FRUITS

Jellies, Jams, and Marmalades

All jams, conserves, and pickles should be preserved in canning jars with two-piece lids. Fill hot jars to within 1/4 inch of the top with hot ingredients. Complete the seal with two-piece lids. Process for 10 minutes in bath of boiling water.

CACTUS PICKLE

2 quarts whole prickly pear fruits
2 cups raw sugar
2/3 cup vinegar
3 ounces red cinnamon candies
1–2 whole cloves (optional)

Remove the skins of the fruits, cut each fruit in half lengthwise, and remove the seeds. Prepare a syrup by mixing the sugar, vinegar, and cinnamon candies in a pot; bring to a boil. Cook pear halves until transparent in the syrup. If you use cloves, put them in a cheesecloth bag so they can be removed before the pickles are put in jars that are equipped with standard canning lids. Process for 15 minutes in a bath of boiling water.

CACTUS-DATE CONSERVE

2 cups thinly sliced prickly pear fruit, seeds removed
18 dates, chopped and pitted
Grated rind from 1 orange
2 thin slices pineapple, cut into small pieces
4 teaspoons lemon juice
$1/2$ cup pineapple juice
$1^1/2$ cups sugar
$1/3$ cup walnuts, broken into pieces

Combine all the ingredients except the walnuts. Cook slowly in a heavy pan until it reaches the desired jam-like consistency. Add the nuts 5 minutes before removing from the heat.

CACTUS PRESERVE

2 quarts whole prickly pear fruit
$1^1/2$ cups raw sugar
$2/3$ cup water
$2^1/2$ tablespoons lemon juice
1 slice orange, $1/4$ inch thick

Remove the skins of the fruit, cut each fruit in half lengthwise, and remove the seeds. Prepare a syrup by mixing the sugar, water, and lemon juice in a pot; bring to a boil. Cook the fruits and the orange slice in the syrup until transparent. Before packing in sterile jars, make sure to remove the orange.

CACTUS-PINEAPPLE MARMALADE

$1/4$ cup pineapple, diced
1 cup prickly pear fruit, peeled, seeded, and diced
$1/2$ cup raw sugar
1 to 2 tablespoons lemon juice

Place the diced pineapple and prickly pear in a pot. Add two times as much water, and bring to boil. Cook, uncovered, until tender. Add the raw sugar and boil vigorously, uncovered, stirring constantly. When the syrup begins to form the texture of jelly, add the lemon juice and boil for one minute more. Pour the mixture into sterilized jelly glasses and seal with paraffin.

The same directions can be followed to prepare Cactus-Lemon Marmalade and Cactus-Orange Marmalade, substituting these fruits for pineapple. The $1/4$ cup of fruit stays the same.

MICROWAVE CACTUS JELLY

$2^1/2$ cups prickly pear cactus juice
1 box powdered pectin
3 tablespoons lemon juice
$3^1/2$ cups raw sugar

In a 3-quart casserole, combine the cactus juice and pectin. Stir until the pectin is dissolved. Microwave on high for 7 to 14 minutes or until boiling, stirring every 3 minutes. Continue to boil for 1 minute.

Add the lemon juice. Gradually stir in the sugar until blended. Microwave on high for 5 to 7 minutes until the mixture returns to boil, stirring every 2 minutes to prevent boiling over. Continue to boil for 2 minutes. Skim the foam from top. Pour the mixture into hot sterilized half-pint jars. Cover with hot sterilized lids and screw bands. Invert the jars and quickly return them to upright position.

JUICES

PRICKLY PEAR PUREE

Strain the raw fruit pulp through a food mill or a medium-fine wire strainer to remove seeds and heavy fibers. Fruit pulp and puree can both be frozen for future use. Simply pack into freezing containers and seal. Thaw before using in a recipe. Seven to ten medium fruits will yield about 1 cup puree.

Indian Fig Juice

Peel the prickly pear fruit and discard the peels. Slice the fruit in half lengthwise and remove the seeds. Place the fruit in one bowl and the seeds in another. When you have about three-quarters of a bowl of seeds, fill the bowl with water and, using your hands, break up the seed clusters so that the pulp clinging to the seeds disperses in the water. Mash the bowl of pure pulp with a potato masher and strain through a mesh strainer or a colander lined with cheesecloth. After the seeds have soaked for a couple of hours, strain off the accumulated liquid and add to it the drained liquid from the mashed pulp. Combine both liquids in a saucepan and simmer for 5 minutes. Pour the juice into clean glass jars and refrigerate. Two dozen tunas yield about 1 quart of juice.

Cactus Juice Cocktail

1 pint chilled cactus juice
1 pint chilled cranberry juice
1 quart chilled ginger ale

Mix the juices in a two-quart pitcher. Add the ginger ale. Dip the rim of drinking glasses in a mixture of lemon juice and water, then in sifted powdered sugar. Pour the cocktail over a couple of ice cubes in the glasses. Serves 2–3.

Cactus Punch

1 pint prickly pear puree
1 pint apple juice
1 pint pineapple-grapefruit juice
1 pint ginger ale or sparkling water (optional)

Combine the prickly pear puree, apple juice, and pineapple-grapefruit juice. Pour the mixture over ice cubes. Add the ginger ale or sparkling water if desired. This recipe can be adjusted for any number of servings by using equal portions of each ingredient. Serves 3–4.

DESSERTS

PRICKLY PEAR SAUCE

A delicious topping for ice cream, custard, or angel food cake.

$^1/_4$ cup raw sugar
1 tablespoon cornstarch
$^1/_8$ teaspoon salt
1 cup prickly pear puree
A few drops almond extract
2 tablespoons lemon juice

Combine the sugar, cornstarch, salt, and puree. Cook, stirring, until slightly thickened and clear, about 5 minutes. Stir in the almond extract and lemon juice and cook a few minutes longer. (For variation, add one 9-ounce can crushed pineapple to the puree. Increase the cornstarch to $1^1/_2$ tablespoons. Makes about 2 cups.) For directions on how to prepare the prickly pear puree, see Juices section of this chapter.

PRICKLY PEAR SALAD RING

1 envelope unflavored gelatin
$^3/_4$ cup water or canned pineapple juice
1 cup prickly pear puree
$^1/_4$ cup raw sugar
$^1/_8$ teaspoon salt
4 tablespoons lime or lemon juice
2 teaspoons finely chopped green onion
$^1/_4$ cup finely chopped celery
1 package (3 ounces) cream cheese
1 small avocado
1 cup drained, diced canned pineapple, or 1 fresh apple, peeled and diced

Soften the gelatin in $^1/_4$ cup of the water or juice. Combine the remaining $^1/_2$ cup liquid with the puree, sugar, and salt; heat to a boil. Dissolve the gelatin in the hot liquid. Stir in the lime or lemon juice, onion, and celery. Cool until the mixture begins to thicken. Cut the cream cheese into small cubes, and stir into the gelatin mixture along with the avocado and pineapple or apple. Turn into a 1-quart mold or 6 individual molds. Chill until firm. Unmold on salad greens. (For a variation, combine the first six ingredients as above. When the mixture begins to congeal, add diced fruits and chopped nuts.) Serves 3–4.

MORE CACTUS TREATS

The following recipes were written by Sandall English and were printed in various articles appearing in the *Arizona Daily Star* and in her book *Fruits of the Desert*.[2,3,4]

PRICKLY PEAR BREAD

1 1/2 cups unbleached white flour
1 1/2 cups whole-wheat flour
3 teaspoons baking powder
1/2 teaspoon sea salt
1/8 teaspoon mace
1/4 cup butter
1/4 cup honey
1 egg
2 tablespoons grated orange rind
3/4 cup ripe prickly pear fruit, peeled, seeded, and cut up
1/4 cup orange juice
1/4 cup prickly pear juice
1/2 cup milk
1/2 teaspoon vanilla
1 cup pecans, chopped

Mix the flours, baking powder, salt, and mace. In separate bowl, cream the butter and honey; beat in the egg. Add the orange rind, prickly pear fruit, orange and prickly pear juices, milk, and vanilla. Add this to the dry ingredients, stirring only until blended. Fold in the nuts. Place in a greased 9-by-5 inch loaf pan. Bake at 350°F for 1 hour or until firm. Makes 1 loaf.

Prickly Pear Whip

1 envelope unflavored gelatin
$1/4$ cup raw sugar
1 cup prickly pear juice
1 cup orange juice
2 tablespoons lemon juice
1 cup plain low-fat yogurt
$1/4$ cup chopped almonds

Mix the gelatin and raw sugar in bowl. Heat the prickly pear juice to a boil in saucepan. Stir the juice into the gelatin mixture until the gelatin is dissolved. Add the orange and lemon juices to the mixture and pour into a bowl to chill. When partially thickened, stir in the yogurt and nuts and beat at low speed or with rotary beater until frothy. Chill until firm. Serves 6.

Prickly Pear Pops (*Palettas* in Spanish)

14 medium prickly pear fruits
1 cup water
2 tablespoons lemon juice concentrate
$1/2$ cup raw sugar

Wash and peel the pears and put them in blender with the water. Add the lemon juice concentrate and raw sugar. Pour the mixture into plastic ice pop makers, or use paper cups and wooden sticks, and freeze. Serves 4.

PRETTY PINK CACTUS-NUT FROZEN YOGURT

This recipe requires the use of an ice cream maker.

1 envelope unflavored gelatin
1 cup prickly pear juice (see recipe in the Juice section)
2 whole eggs, separated
1 (32-ounce) container unflavored yogurt
1 cup raw sugar, divided
2 tablespoons vanilla
½ cup toasted, chopped almonds

Combine the gelatin and juice. Let stand for about 5 minutes, then heat to a boil, stirring until the gelatin completely dissolves. Cool for about 5 minutes. Beat the egg yolks lightly with wire wisk; add the yogurt and ¾ cup raw sugar and beat until smooth. Beat in the gelatin mixture and vanilla.

Beat the egg whites until soft peaks form. Gradually beat in the remaining ¼ cup raw sugar, beating until firm. Fold into the yogurt mixture. Add more sugar to taste, if desired. Pour the mixture into an ice cream freezer can and refrigerate.

Coarsely chop the almonds, place in an ungreased heavy skillet, and brown, stirring occasionally. Cool slightly and add to the yogurt mixture, stirring well. Assemble the ice cream maker and proceed according to the manufacturer's directions. Makes about 1½ quarts.

PRICKLY PEAR FLIP

4 ice cubes
2 ounces prickly pear juice, chilled
2 ounces pineapple juice, chilled
2 teaspoons lemon juice
2 teaspoons honey (or raw sugar) to taste
½ cup papaya cubes, peeled and seeded
½ cup evaporated skim milk

In a blender, combine all the ingredients; blend until smooth. Pour the mixture into two 8-ounce glasses and serve at once. Serves 2.

Cactus Candy

7 or 8 washed prickly pears
2 envelopes unflavored gelatin
1½ cup water
2 cups raw sugar
⅛ teaspoon salt
Powdered sugar, for coating

Place the prickly pears in a blender with 1 cup water and liquefy. Strain the juice through layers of cheesecloth, and measure out 1 cup juice. Soften the gelatin with ½ cup water. Bring the strained prickly pear juice, raw sugar, and salt to a boil, add the gelatin to the hot juice, and stir until dissolved. Boil slowly for 10 minutes.

Pour the mixture into an 8-inch square pan. Allow it to set for at least 12 hours. Cut the candy into small squares and roll them in powdered sugar. Serves 3–4.

Prickly Pear Suppliers

Below is a list of key natural product, food, and dietary supplement companies in the U.S. marketplace. These companies retail the prickly pear pads, fruits, flowers, or a combination of the three as part of an existing product line assortment.

For the most up-to-date resource information please visit my Web site at **www.cactusmedicine.com**

NUTRITIONAL SUPPLEMENTS

Aztec Ltd.
P.O. Box 30, Ponteland
Newcastle Upon Tyne NE20 9YL
United Kingdom
001-44-1670-1513060
www.nopalaztec.com
Products: Nopal cactus capsules, liquid concentrate, and dehydrated powders

Bio Serae
N 1 Avenue de la Preulihe
Parc Technologique du Lauragais
11150 Bram, France
011-33-4-68-76-76-20
www.neopuntia.com
Products: Standardized fat binder that prevents fat from being absorbed in the lower intestine

Cactu Life
P.O. Box 349
Corona Del Mar, CA 92625
949-640-8991

www.cactulife.com
Products: Encapsulated prickly pear pad products for weight loss, diabetes, cholesterol, and general immune system

Desert Bloom International
3255 Wilshire Blvd., Ste. 1708
Los Angeles, CA 90010
213-384-0500
www.nopaljuice.com
Products: Nopal Extract nutritional supplements

Herbamed Ltd.
Kiryat Weizmann Science
Industrial Park
Rehovot, Israel
www.herbamed.co.il/
Product: Prostacal

HVL Douglas Laboratories
600 Boyce Rd.
Pittsburgh, PA 15205-9742
412-494-0122
www.douglaslabs.com
Products: Nopal Leaf Vegicaps, Formula VRC (Natural Immune Support)

Nature's Sunshine Products, Inc.
75 E. 1700 South
Provo, UT 84606
801-342-4300
www.naturessunshine.com
Products: Nopal and SugarReg

Nature's Way
10 Mountain Springs Parkway
Springville, Utah 84663
801-489-1500
www.naturesway.com
Products: Opuntia Prickly Pear Flowers, Blood Sugar Formula, ProstActive

Neem Tree Farms
601 Southwood Cv.
Brandon, FL 33511-7134
813-661-8873
www.neemtreefarms.com
Products: USDA certified organic nopal

Nutraceutical International Corporation
1400 Kearns Blvd., 2nd Fl.
Park City, UT 84060
800-669-8877
www.nutraceutical.com
Products: Blood Sugar Defense and Peaceful Planet: The Supreme
Meal

Perfect Equation, Inc.
2460 Coral St.
Vista, CA 92081
760-599-6079
www.perfectequation.net
Products: HPF (Hangover Prevention Formula), Prepair

Solgar Vitamin and Herb
500 Willow Tree Rd.
Leonia, NJ 07605
877-765-4274
www.solgar.com
Products: Saw Palmetto Pygeum Lycopene Complex Vegetable Capsules

Swanson Health Products
Customer Care
P.O. Box 2803
Fargo, ND 58108-2803
800-603-3198
www.swansonvitamins.com
Products: NeOpuntia, Nopal Cactus Powder, and Nopal signature
brand

FOOD & BEVERAGE INDUSTRY MANUFACTURERS (PACKAGED FOODS)

Arizona Cactus Ranch

P.O. Box 8
Green Valley, AZ 85622
800-582-9903
www.arizonacactusranch.com
Products: Prickly Pear Nectar, Cactus Fruit Salsa, Prickly Pear Fruit
Spread, Prickly Pear Topping
Note: At the time of publication, cactus provided by Arizona Cactus
Ranch is being used in scientific research to determine its potential in
the prevention of different types of cancer.

Cactus Candy Co.

3010 N 24th St.
Phoenix, AZ 85016-7816
602-956-4833
www.cactuscandy.com
Products: Cactus Candy, Prickly Pear Syrup, Cactus Jelly, Prickly
Pear Marmalade

Cheri's Desert Harvest

1840 E Winsett
Tucson, AZ 85719-6548
800-743-1141
www.cherisdesertharvest.com
Products: Cactus Apple Jelly, Prickly Pear Jelly, Cactus Honey,
Cactus Marmalade, Cactus Chocolates, Prickly Pear Cactus Candy,
Prickly Pear Cactus Syrup

Desert Rose Foods, Inc.

P.O. Box 28247
Scottsdale, AZ 85255
800-937-2572
www.desertrosefoods.biz
Products: Cactus Catsup, Cactus Candy

Dona Maria, a line of Grupo Herdez, S.A. de C.V.
Corporativo Cinco S.A. de C.V.
Monte Pelvoux No. 125
Col. Lomas de Chapultepec
C.P. 11000 Mexico, D.F.
011-52-55-5201-5655
www.grupoherdez.com.mx
Product: Tender Cactus

Embasa Foods
(A subsidiary of Authentic Specialty Foods, Inc.)
4340 Eucalyptus Ave.
Chino, CA 91710-9705
888-236-2272
www.embasa.com
Product: Sliced Nopalitos

Goya Foods, Inc.
100 Seaview Dr.
Secaucus, NJ 07094
201-348-4900
www.goyafoods.com
Products: Nopalitos

Royal Crown Foods
780 Epperson Dr.
City of Industry, CA 91748
626-854-8080
www.mexgrocer.com
Product: Royal Crown Nopalitos

Vilore Foods Company, Inc.
8220 San Lorenzo Dr.
Laredo, TX 78045
956-726-3633
www.vilore.com
Product: La Costeña Nopalitos

COSMETICS MANUFACTURERS

Prickly pear cactus cosmetics are a new and emerging category. There are many boutique companies that offer prickly pear cosmetics within their existing product lines. It is estimated that there are hundreds of companies selling a variety of prickly pear items for cosmetic or topical healing application. These products include shampoos, conditioners, gels, and essential oils.

Arizona Natural Resources, Inc.
2525 E Beardsley Rd.
Phoenix, AZ 85050-1322
602-569-6900
www.arizonanaturalresources.com
Products: Prickly Pear Moisturizing Body Wash, Prickly Pear Hand and Body Lotion, Prickly Pear Foaming Milk Bath

Cactus Juice
(Safe Solutions, Inc.)
1007 North Cactus Tr.
Seymour, TX 76380
940-888-5222
www.cactusjuicetm.com
Products: Prickly pear–based sun/skin/outdoor protection, Miracle Gel, Desert Spring Total Body Lotion, Skin and Outdoor Protectant Spray

Nanny's Best
2928 CR 409
Hamilton, TX 76531-3024
254-386-3622
www.nannysbest.com
Products: Paws and Claws, All Purpose Cleaner, Moisturizer, Shampoo, Insect Spray, Animal Shampoo

Santa Fe Soap Co.
369 Montezuma Ave., #167
Santa Fe, NM 87501
888-762-7227
www.santafesoap.com
Products: Cactus Soap

Totally You
2700 Business Center Blvd.
Melbourne, FL 32940
800-254-5900
www.totallyyou.com
Products: Sea Clay Prickly Pear Conditioner, Sea Clay Prickly Pear Shampoo, Sea Clay Prickly Pear Styling Gel

Cactus Mary's
3219 Altura Ave.
El Paso, TX 79930-4429
915-565-7825
www.cactusmary.com
Product: Prickly Pear Soap

ALCOHOL DISTRIBUTORS

Aguirre Tequila Imports
1225 Santo Domingo Ave.
Duarte, CA 91010
626-359-1913
www.lajaula.com.mx
Product: El Gran Tunal (hard alcohol from the prickly pear fruit), Vino Hacienda la Juala (Prickly Pear Fruit Wine), Copil (prickly pear fruit liqueur)

Herbal Education and Natural Product Services

Below are some of the most prominent institutions working in the field of herbal education and medical herbalism research. I have also included contact information for my own company, NutraConsulting, which works to expand the availability and success of nutraceuticals in the marketplace.

NutraConsulting

333 River St., Ste. 650
Hoboken, NJ 07030
551-655-8976
www.nutraconsulting.com

NutraConsulting was founded in 2002 by author Ran Knishinsky. Their specialty is the fulfillment of strategic research, new product development, supply-chain management, and marketing services for underdeveloped, underutilized, or undiscovered botanicals, nutraceuticals, and mineral clay products. They identify those products with keen potential to be retailed as dietary supplements or natural product SKU's inside and outside the healthy foods channel.

American Botanical Council

6200 Manor Rd.
Austin, TX 78723
www.herbalgram.org

The American Botanical Council is a nonprofit education and research organization, and a copublisher, with the Herb Research Foundation, of *HerbalGram*. In addition, they publish booklets on herbs and reprints of scientific articles.

The American Herbalists Guild
1931 Gaddis Rd.
Canton, GA 30115
770-751-6021
www.americanherbalistguild.com
The American Herbalists Guild's members range from clinical practitioners to ethnobotanists who are committed to the advancing field
of medical herbalism. They can provide a directory of schools and
teachers.

American Herbal Pharmacopoeia
P.O. Box 66809
Scotts Valley, CA 95067
831-461-6318
www.herbal-ahp.org
The American Herbal Pharmacopoeia promotes the art and science
of healing, supplying knowledge of herbal medicine to professionals
and laypersons in the health care field. They also publish herbal
monographs.

Association of Natural Medicine Pharmacists (ANMP)
P.O. Box 150727
San Rafael, CA 94915
415-479-1512
www.anmp.org
The Association of Natural Medicine Pharmacists raises awareness
of botanical medicine and provides educational materials on natural
medicines to practicing pharmacists.

Herb Research Foundation
4140 15th St.
Boulder, CO 80302
303-449-2265
www.herbs.org
The Herb Research Foundation provides research materials for
consumers, physicians, pharmacists, scientists, and the health food
industry. They are copublishers, with the American Botanical
Council, of *HerbalGram*.

North American Institute of Medical Herbalism

P.O. Box 20512
Boulder, CO 80308
www.medherb.com

The North American Institute of Medical Herbalism provides links to medical information relevant to medicinal herbs or herbalism practiced in a clinical setting. It publishes a quarterly newsletter, *Medical Herbalism,* written primarily for practitioners of botanical medicine.

General Resources for Diabetes and Heart Disease

For further information on diabetes and heart disease, in addition to professional referrals, contact these institutions:

American Association of Diabetes Educators (AADE)

100 West Monroe St., Ste. 400
Chicago, IL 60603
800-338-3633
www.aadenet.org

The American Association of Diabetes Educators is dedicated to advancing the role of the diabetes educator and improving the quality of diabetes education and care.

American Association of Naturopathic Physicians

3201 New Mexico Ave., NW Ste. 350
Washington, DC 20016
866-538-2267
www.naturopathic.org

The American Association of Naturopathic Physicians provides referrals to a nationwide network of accredited or licensed practitioners. It publishes a quarterly letter for both professionals and the general public.

American Diabetes Association (ADA)

ADA National Service Center
ATTN: National Call Center
1701 North Beauregard St.
Alexandria, VA 22311
800-Diabetes (800-342-2383)
www.diabetes.org

The American Diabetes Association's mission is to prevent and cure diabetes and to improve the lives of all people affected by diabetes.

American Dietetic Association

120 S. Riverside Plaza, Ste. 2000
Chicago, IL 60606
800-877-1600
www.eatright.org
The American Dietetic Association promotes optimal nutrition and well-being for all people by advocating for its members.

American Heart Association

7272 Greenville Ave
Dallas, TX 75231
800-242-8721
www.americanheart.org
The American Heart Association is a nonprofit health agency devoted to the fight against heart disease, stroke, and other cardiovascular illnesses.

American Holistic Medical Association

12101 Menaul Blvd., NE, Ste. C
Albuquerque, NM 87112
505-292-7788
www.holisticmedicine.org
The American Holistic Medical Association is an organization of holistic doctors and doctors of osteopathy who practice integrated medicine and can provide referrals to practitioners in your area.

Centers for Disease Control and Prevention

National Center for Chronic Disease Prevention and Health Promotion
1600 Clifton Rd.
Atlanta, GA 30333
800-311-3435
www.cdc.gov
Reduces the burden of diabetes in the United States by planning, coordinating, and evaluating federal efforts to translate promising results of diabetes research into widespread clinical and public health practice.

International Diabetes Center (IDC)

3800 Park Nicollet Blvd.
Minneapolis, MN 55416
888-825-6315
www.parknicollet.com/diabetes

The International Diabetes Center partners with health care providers throughout the world to promote better care for persons with diabetes. They offer educational programs for people with diabetes, and training programs for health care professionals that focus on team management of diabetes.

International Diabetes Federation (IDF)

19 Avenue Emile De Mot, B-1000
Brussels, Belgium
011-322-538-55-11
011-322-538-51-14 (fax)
www.idf.org

The IDF is an alliance of 183 national diabetes associations in 142 countries. The aim of the IDF is to bring together people all over the world who are concerned with diabetes, through their professional or personal lives, and to use their combined strengths to further the cause of the person with diabetes.

Joslin Diabetes Center

1 Joslin Pl.
Boston, MA 02215
617-732-2415
www.joslin.org

Joslin Diabetes Center is an international leader in diabetes research, treatment, and patient and professional education, and was established in 1898 in Boston, affiliated with Harvard Medical School.

Juvenile Diabetes Research Foundation (JDRF)

120 Wall St.
New York, NY 10005
800-JDF-CURE
www.jdf.org

The JDRF was founded in 1970 by parents of children with diabetes. Their mission: to find a cure for diabetes and its complications through the support of research. JDRF is organized on a business-world model, a focus that enables the organization to provide at least 80 cents of every dollar raised to research and education about research.

National Diabetes Information Clearinghouse (NDIC)

1 Information Way
Bethesda, MD 20892-3560
www.diabetes.niddk.nih.gov

The National Diabetes Information Clearinghouse is a service of the NIDDK designed to increase knowledge and understanding about diabetes among patients and their families, healthcare professionals, and the public.

The National Institute of Diabetes and Digestive and Kidney Diseases (NIDDK)

Office of Communications and Public Liaison, NIDDK, NIH
Bldg. 31, Rm. 9A04 Center Dr., MSC 2560
Bethesda, MD 20892-2560
www.niddk.nih.gov

In its mission to conduct and support research on kidney, urologic, hematologic, digestive, metabolic, and endocrine diseases, as well as on diabetes and nutrition, the NIDDK also provides a wealth of easy-to-read health information for the public.

Notes

Chapter 1: Cactus Medicine

1. Richard Stephen Felger and Mary Beck Moser, *People of the Desert and Sea: Ethnobotany of the Seri Indians* (Tucson: University of Arizona Press, 1985), 109.
2. Kathleen Walker, "The Cactus Cookers: Serving up the Fruit of the Desert," *Arizona Highways* (Feb 1996): 23–25.
3. Ibid.
4. Mark Blumenthal, "Herbal Update: Testing Botanicals," *Whole Foods* 20, no. 7 (1997): 52.
5. Ibid.
6. Robert A. DiSilvestro, "Flavonoids as Antioxidants" in Ira Wolinsky and James F. Hickson, ed., *Handbook of Nutraceuticals and Functional Foods* (Boca Raton, Fla.: CRC Press, LLC, 2001), 127–42.
7. L. Bravo, "Polyphenols: Chemistry, Dietary Sources, Metabolism, and Nutritional Significance," *Nutrition Review* 56, no. 11 (Nov 1998): 317–33.
8. Z. Min and X. Peigen, "Quantitative Analysis of the Active Constituents in Green Tea. *Phytotherapy Research* 5 (1991): 239–40.
9. E. L. Pautler, J. A. Maga, and C. Tengerdy, "A Pharmacologically Potent Natural Product in the Bovine Retina," *Experimental Eye Research* 42 (1986): 285–88.
10. Murray, *The Healing Power of Herbs,* 54.
11. B. Schwitters and Jacques Masquelier, "OPC in Practice: Biflavanols and Their Application," Alfa Omega, Rome (1993)," in Michael T. Murray, *The Healing Power of Herbs,* 186.
12. M. M. Kanter, "Free Radicals and Exercise: Effects of Nutritional Antioxidant Supplementation," *Exercise Sports Science Review* 23 (1995): 375–97.
13. Lisa Schofield, "The ABC's of OPC's," *Vitamin Retailer* 4, no. 11 (Nov 1997): 18–24.
14. Amanda Spake, "Tea Time," *US News & World Report* 132, no. 17, 20 May 2002, p. 52.

15. Ibid.

16. C. Ghiringhelli, F. Gregoratti, and F. Marastoni, "Capillarotropic Action of Anthocyanosides in High Dosage in Phlebopathic Statis," *Minerva Cardioangiologica* 26 (1978): 255–76.

17. Michael T. Murray, *The Healing Power of Herbs: The Enlightened Person's Guide to the Wonders of Medicinal Plants* (Rocklin, Calif.: Prima Publishing, 1995), 186.

18. DiSilvestro, "Flavonoids as Antioxidants," 127–42.

19. Ibid.

20. B. M. Babior, "The Respiratory Burst Oxidase," *Current Opinion Hematol* 2 (1995): 55–60.

21. J. P. Kehrer, "Free Radicals as Mediators of Tissue Injury and Disease," *Critical Reviews in Toxicology* 23 (1993): 21–48.

22. O. A. Parks and D. N. Granger, "Xanthine Oxidase: Biochemistry, Distribution, and Psychology," *Acta Physiologica Scandinavica* 5485 (1986): 87–99.

23. Y. Pingzhang, Z. Jinying, et al., "Experimental Studies of the Inhibitory Effects of Green Tea Catechin on Mice Large Intestinal Cancers Induced by 1, 2–dinethylhydrazine," *Cancer Letters* 79 (1994): 33–38.

24. Murray, *The Healing Power of Herbs,* 16–17.

25. C. Ho, et al., "Antioxidative Effect of Polyphenol Extract Prepared from Various Chinese Teas," *Preventative Medicine* 21 (1992): 4050–52.

26. Albert I. Wertheimer, Richard Levy, and Thomas W. O'Connor, "Too Many Drugs? The Clinical and Economic Value of Incremental Innovations," *Investing in Health: The Social and Economic Benefits of Health Care Innovation* 14 (2001): 77–118.

27. Burton Goldberg Group, *Alternative Medicine, the Definitive Guide* (Puyallup, Wash.: Future Medicine Publishing, Inc., 1993), 254.

28. N. R. Farnsworth, et al., "Medicinal Plants in Therapy," *Bulletin of the World Health Organization* 63, no. 6 (1985): 965–81. Reprinted in *Alternative Medicine, the Definitive Guide.*

29. Ran Knishinsky, *The Prozac Alternative,* (Rochester, Vt.: Healing Arts Press, 1998), 9.

30. Burton Goldberg Group, *Alternative Medicine,* 254–55.

31. Ibid.

32. Ibid.

33. Ibid.

Chapter 2: What Is a Cactus?

1. W. Hubert Earle, *Cacti of the Southwest* (Tempe, Ariz.: Rancho Arryo, 1980): 1–5.
2. William G. McGinnies, *Discovering the Desert* (Tucson: The University of Arizona Press, 1981): 186.
3. Earle, *Cacti of the Southwest,* 1–5.
4. Reg. Manning, *What Kinda Cactus Izzat?* (Phoenix: Reganson Cartoon Books, 1964), 3.
5. Benson Lyman, *The Cacti of Arizona,* (Tucson: University of Arizona Press, 1984), 29.
6. Manning, *What Kinda Cactus Izzat?,* 5.
7. McGinnies, *Discovering the Desert,* 17–25
8. Ibid.
9. Edward Abbey and the Editors of Time-Life Books, *Cactus Country* (New York: Time Life Books, 1973), 95.

Chapter 3: The Healing Parts of the Prickly Pear Cactus

1. Kazeminy, "Report of Laboratory Analysis - Mineral" conducted by Irvine Analytical Laboratories, Incorporated on samples of Cactulife's dehydrated *Opuntia streptacantha*. 30 November 1995.
2. Kazeminy, "Report of Laboratory Analysis - Amino Acid Profile" conducted by Irvine Analytical Laboratories, Incorporated on samples of Cactulife's dehydrated *Opuntia streptacantha*. 7 July 1994.
3. Karen Shapiro and William C. Gong, "Use of Herbal Products for Diabetes by Latinos," *Journal of the American Pharmaceutical Association,* 42, no. 2 (Mar/Apr 2002): 278–82.
4. Ibid.
5. Alberto C. Frati-Munari, Blanca E. Gordillo, Perla Altamirano, and C. Raul Ariza, "Hypoglycemic Effect of *Opuntia streptacantha* Lemaire in NIDDM," *Diabetes Care* 2, No. 1 (Jan 1998): 63–66.
6. Sandall English, "Cacti for Connoisseurs," *The Arizona Daily Star,* 18 May 1994.
7. Walker, "The Cactus Cookers," 23–25.

Chapter 4: The Cactus-Diabetes Connection

1. "Cactus Lowers Blood Glucose Levels," *Science News* 133, no. 4, (Jan 1988).
2. R. Ibanez-Camacho, M. Meckes-Lozoya, and V. Mellado-Campos, "The Hypoglycemic Effect of *Opuntia streptacantha* Studied in

Different Animal Experimental Models," *Journal of Ethnopharmacology* 7 (1983): 175–81.

3. A. C. Frati-Munari, A. Yever-Garces, M. Becerril, S. Isals, R. Ariza, "Studies on the Mechanism of 'Hypoglycemic' Effect of Nopal (*Opuntia* sp.)", *Archivos de Investigacion. Medica (Mexico)* 18 (1987): 7–12.

4. Frati-Munari, Gordillo, Altamirano, and Ariza, "Hypoglycemic Effect of *Opuntia streptacantha* Lemaire in NIDDM," 63–66.

5. A. C. Frati-Munari, J. A. Fernandez-Harp, M. Becerril, A. Chavez-Negrete, M. Banales-Ham, "Decrease in Serum Lipds, Glycemia and Body Weight by *Plantago psyllium* in Obese and Diabetic Patients," *Archivos de Investigacion Medica (Mexico)* 14 (1983): 259–68.

6. David Cameron-Smith and Gregory R. Collier, "Dietary Fiber and Glucose Metabolism and Diabetes," in *Handbook of Dietary Fiber* (New York: Marcel Dekker, Inc., 2001), 107–21.

7. M. Meckes-Lozyoa and R. Roman-Ramos, "*Opuntia streptacantha*: A Coadjutor in the Treatment of Diabetes Mellitus," *American Journal of Chinese Medicine* 14, nos. 3–4 (1986): 116–18.

8. Ibanez-Camacho, et al., "The Hypoglycemic Effect Of *Opuntia streptacantha* Studied in Different Animal Experimental Models," 175–81.

9. Ibid.

10. R. Roman-Ramos, J. L. Flores-Saenz, and F. J. Alarcon-Aguilar, "Anti-hyperglycemic Effect of Some Edible Plants," *Journal of Ethnopharamacology* 48 (1995): 25–32.

11. A. C. Frati-Munari, B. E. Gordollo, P. Altamirano, C. R. Ariza, R. Cortes-Franco, A. Chavez-Negrete, S. Islas-Andrade, "Influence of Nopal Intake Upon Fasting Glycemia in Type II Diabetics and Healthy Subjects," *Archivos de Investigacion Medica (Mexico)* 22, no. 1 (1991): 51–56.

12. A. C. Frati-Munari, J. A. Fernandez-Harp, H. De la Riva, R. Ariza-Andraca, and M.C. Torres, "Effects of Nopal (*Opuntia* sp.) on Serum Lipids, Glycemia and Body Weight," *Archivos de Investigacion Medica (Mexico)* 14 (1983): 117–25.

13. A. C. Frati-Munari, J. A. Fernandez-Harp, M. Banales-Ham, and C. R. Ariza-Andraca, "Decreased Blood Glucose and Insulin by Nopal (*Opuntia* sp.)," *Archivos de Investigacion Medica (Mexico)* 14 (1983): 269–73.

14. M. Meckes-Lozyoa and R. Ibanez-Camacho, "Hypoglycemic Activity of *Opuntia Streptacantha* Throughout Its Annual Cycle," *American Journal of Chinese Medicine* 17, nos. 3–4 (1989): 221–24.

15. A. C. Frati, N. Diaz Xilotl, P. Altamirano, R. Ariza, R. Lopez-Lesema, R, "The Effect of Two Sequential Doses of *Opuntia Streptacantha* upon Glycemia," *Archivos de Investigacion Medica (Mexico)* 22, nos. 3–4 (1991): 333–36.

16. A. C. Frati-Munari, L. M. Del Valle-Martinez, C. R. Ariza-Andraca, S. Isals-Andrade, A. Chavez-Negrete, "Hypoglycemic Action of Different Doses of Nopal (*Opuntia streptacantha* Lemaire) in Patients with Type II Diabetes Mellitus," *Archivos de Investigaccion Medica (Mexico)*, 20, no. 2 (1989): 197–201.

17. A. C. Frati-Munari, Gil. U. Rios, C. R. Ariza-Andraca, S. Islas-Andrade, R. Lopez-Ledesma, "Duration of the Hypoglycemic Action of *Opuntia streptacantha*," *Archivos de Investigaccion Medica (Mexico)*, 20, no. 4 (1989): 297–300.

18. A. C. Frati-Munari, R. Licona-Quesada, C. R. Araiza-Andraca, R. Lopez-Ledesma, A. Chavez-Negrete, "Activity of *Opuntia streptacantha* in Healthy Individuals with Induced Hyperglycemia," *Archivos de Investigacion Medica (Mexico)* 21, no. 2 (1990): 99–102.

19. A. C. Frati-Munari, E. Altamirano-Bustamente, N. Rodriguez-Barcenas, R. Ariza-Andraca, R. Lopez-Ledesma, "Hypoglycemic Action of *Opuntia streptacantha* Lemaire: Study Using Raw Extracts," *Archivos de Investigacion Medica (Mexico)* 20, no. 4 (1989): 321–25.

20. A. C. Frati-Munari, C. Leon, R. Ariza-Andraca, M.B. Banales-Ham, R. Lopez-Ledesma, S. Lozoya, "Effect of a Dehydrated Extract of Nopal *(Opuntia ficus-indica)* on Blood Glucose," *Archivos de Investigacion Medica (Mexico)*, 20, no. 3 (1989): 211–16.

21. A.C. Frati, E. Jiminez, and C.R. Ariza, "Hypoglycemic Effect of *Opuntia ficus-indica* in Non Insulin-dependent Diabetes Mellitus Patients," *Phytotherapy Research* 4, no. 5 (1990): 195–97.

22. A. C. Frati-Munari, O. Vera Lastra, C. R. Ariza Andraca, "Evaluation of Nopal Capsules in Diabetes Mellitus," *Gaceta Medica de Mexico*, 128, No. 4 (1992): 431–36.

23. A. Trejo-Gonzalez, G. Gabriel-Ortiz, A. M. Puebla-Perez, M. D. Huizar-Contrera, M. R. Munguia-Mazariegos, S. Meja-Arreguin, E.

Calva, "A Purified Extract from Prickly Pear Cactus *(Opuntia fuliginosa)* Controls Experimentally Induced Diabetes in Rats," *Journal of Ethnopharamacology* 55, no. 1 (Dec 1996): 27–33.

24. Jane Erickson, "Eating Prickly Pear Can Cut 'Bad' Cholesterol, UA Scientist Says," *Arizona Daily Star,* 2 February 1992.

25. Marina Perfumi and Rosalia Tacconi, "Antihyperglycemic Effect of Fresh *Opuntia Dilleni* Fruit from Tenerife (Canary Islands)," *International Journal of Pharmacognosy* 34, no. 1 (1996): 41–47.

Chapter 5: The Cactus-Cholesterol Connection

1. Erickson, "Eating Prickly Pear Can Cut 'Bad' Cholesterol, UA Scientist Says."

2. Maria Luz Fernandez, "Pectin: Composition, Chemistry, Physicochemical Properties, Food Applications, and Physiological Effects," in Susan Sungsoo and Mark L. Dreher, ed., *Handbook of Dietary Fiber,* (New York: Marcel Dekker, Inc., 2001), 583–601.

3. M. L. Fernandez, Emme C. K. Lin, Augusto Trejo, and D. J. McNamara, "Prickly Pear *(Opuntia* sp.) Pectin Alters Hepatic Cholesterol Metabolism without Affecting Cholesterol Absorption in Guinea Pigs Fed a Hypercholesterolemic Diet," *The Journal of Nutrition* 124 (1994): 817–24.

4. M. L. Fernandez, Emme C. K. Lin, Augusto Trejo, and D. J. McNamara, "Prickly Pear *(Opuntia* sp.) Pectin Reverses Low Density Lipoprotein Receptor Suppression Induced by a Hypercholesterolemic Diet in Guinea Pigs," *The Journal of Nutrition* 122 (1992): 2330–40.

5. M. L. Fernandez, Emme C. K. Lin, Augusto Trejo, and D. J. McNamara, "Pectin Isolated from Prickly Pear *(Opuntia* sp.) Modifies Low Density Lipoprotein Metabolism in Cholesterol-Fed Guinea Pigs," *The Journal of Nutrition* 120 (1990): 1283–90.

6. Ibid.

7. M. L. Fernandez, Dong Ming Sun, Mark A. Tosca, and Donald J. McNamara, "Citrus Pectin and Cholesterol Interact to Regulate Hepatic Cholesterol Homeostasis and Lipoprotein Metabolism A Dose-Response Study in Guinea Pigs," *The American Journal of Clinical Nutrition,* 59 (1994): 669–878.

8. Fernandez, Lin, Trejo, and McNamara, "Prickly Pear *(Opuntia* sp.) Pectin Reverses Low Density Lipoprotein Receptor Suppression Induced by a Hypercholesterolemic Diet in Guinea Pigs," 2330–40.

9. B. Frei, R. Strocker, and B. N. Ames, "Small Molecule Antioxidant Defenses in Human Extracellular fluids," 23–45, in Jeong-Chae Lee, et al., "Effects of Cactus and Ginger Extracts as Dietary Antioxidants on Reactive Oxidant and Plasma Lipid Level," Food Science and Biotechnology 9, no. 2 (2000).

10. Jeong-Chae Lee and Kye-Taek Lim, "Effects of Cactus and Ginger Extracts as Dietary Antioxidants on Reactive Oxidant and Plasma Lipid Level," *Food Science and Biotechnology* 9, no. 2 (2000): 83–88.

11. Ibid.

12. J. Regnstrom, J. Nilsson, P. Tornvail, C. Landou, and A. Hamsten, "Susceptibility to Low-density Lipoprotein Oxidation and Coronary Atherosclerosis in Man," *Lancet* 339 (1992): 1183–86, in Lee, Jeong-Chae, et. al.

13. M. Torres, R. Posadas, J. Zamora, A. Trejo, S. Ichazo, G. Cardoso, C. Posadas, "Efficacy and Safety of Prickly Pear Pectin (*Opuntia* sp.) in Patients with Mild Hypercholesterolemia. XII International Symposium on Drugs Affecting Lipid Metabolism," Houston (1995): 153.

14. Ibid.

15. J. J. Cerda, S. J. Normann, M. P. Sullivan, C. W. Burgin, F. L. Robbins, S. Vathada, P. Leelachaikul, "Inhibition of Atherosclerosis by Dietary Pectin in Microswine with Sustained Hypercholesterolemia," *Circulation* 89 (1994): 1247–53, in Fernandez, "Pectin: Composition, Chemistry, Physicochemical Properties, Food Applications, and Physiological Effects."

16. Fernandez, "Pectin: Composition, Chemistry, Physicochemical Properties, Food Applications, and Physiological Effects," 583–601.

17. M. Kay, A. S. Truswell, "Effect of Citrus Pectin on Blood Lipids and Fecal Steroid Excretion in Man," *American Journal of Clinical Nutrition* 30 (1977): 171–75.

18. T. A. Miettinen, S. Tarpila, "Effect of Pectin on Serum Cholesterol, Fecal Bile Acids and Biliary Lipids in Normolipidemic and Hyperlipidemic Individuals," *Clinica Chimica Acta: International Journal of Clinical Chemistry* 79 (1977): 471–77.

19. D. J. A. Jenkins, A. R. Leeds, C. Newton, J. H. Cummings, "Effect of Pectin, Guar Gum and Wheat Fibre on Serum Cholesterol," *Lancet* 1 (1975): 1116–17.

20. Maria Luz Fernandez, "Pectin: Composition, Chemistry, Physicochemical Properties, Food Applications, and Physiological Effects," 596.

Chapter 6: Other Benefits of and Treatments Using Prickly Pear Cactus

1. Walker, "The Cactus Cookers," 23–25.
2. Michael Moore, *Medicinal Plants of the Desert and Canyon West,* (Santa Fe: Museum of New Mexico Press, 1989): 89–91.
3. Julia Frances Morton, *Atlas of Medicinal Plants of Middle America: Bahamas to Yucatan* (Springfield, Ill.: Charles C. Thomas Publisher, 1981): 605–6.
4. Ibid.
5. Ibid., 607.
6. E. H. Park and M. J. Chun, "Wound Healing Activity of *Opuntia ficus-indica,*" *Fitoterapia* 2, no. 2 (Feb 2001): 165–67.
7. E. H. Park, J. H. Kahng, E. A. Paek, "Studies on the Pharmacological Actions of Cactus: Indentification of Its Anti-inflammatory Effect," *Archives of Pharmacal Research* 21 (Feb 1998): 30–34.
8. Douglas Schar, "The Workout Herb," *Prevention* (Apr 2003): 55.
9. D. Palevitch, G. Earon, and I. Levin, "Treatment of Benign Prostatic Hypertrophy with *Opuntia ficus-indica* (L.) Miller," *Journal of Herbs, Spices & Medicinal Plants,* 2 no. 1 (1993): 45–49.
10. B. Giuseppe, F. Carimi, and P. Inglese, "Past and Present Role of the Indian-fig Prickly-pear *(Opuntia ficus-indica (L.) Miller,* Cactaceae) in the Agriculture of Sicily," *Economic Botany,* 46 (1992): 10–20.
11. L. Boulos, *Medicinal Plants of Northern Africa* (Algonac, Mich.: Reference Publications, Inc., 1983): 40.
12. *British Herbal Pharmacopoeia* (West York, England: The British Herbal Medicine Association, 1983): 255.
13. Moore, *Medicinal Plants of the Desert and Canyon West,* 89–91.
14. Adi Jonas, Gennady Rosen, Daniel Krapt William Bitterman, Ishak Neeman, "Cactus Flower Extracts May Prove Beneficial in Benign Prostatic Hyperplasia due to Inhibition of 5alpha Activity, Aromatase Activity and Lipid Peroxidation," *Urological Research* 26 (1998): 265–70.
15. Morton, *Atlas of Medicinal Plants of Middle America,* 608.
16. A. Ahmad, J. Davies, S. Randall, and G. R. B. Skinner, "Antiviral Properties of Extract of *Opuntia streptacantha,*" *Antiviral Research* 30 (1996): 75–85.

17. Morton, *Atlas of Medicinal Plants of Middle America*, 608–9.
18. Daniel E. Moerman, "Medicinal Plants of Native America, Research Reports in Ethnobotany," contribution 2, *University of Michigan Museum of Anthropology, Technical Reports* 19 (1986): 314.
19. Ibid.
20. Ibid.

Chapter 7: Application and Dosage of Prickly Pear Cactus

1. M. G. Hertog, et al., "Dietary Antioxidant Flavonoids and Risk of Coronary Heart Disease: The Zutphen Elderly Study," *Lancet* 342 (1993): 1007–11, in Michael T. Murray's *The Healing Power of Herbs,* 190.

Chapter 8: Picking and Preparing the Prickly Pear

1. Walker, "The Cactus Cookers," 23–25.
2. M. D. White, B. Linda, and Steven Foster, *The Herbal Drugstore: The Best Natural Alternatives to Over-the-Counter and Prescription Medicines!* (New York: Rodale Press, 2000), 22.
3. Hodgson, W., *Edible Native and Naturalized Plants of the Sonoran Desert North of Mexico* (Tempe: Arizona State University, 1985), 246.

Chapter 9: Cactus Cooking

1. The following recipes in this chapter were provided by the Pima County Office, Arizona Cooperative Extension, U.S. Department of Agriculture (Tucson: The University of Arizona), unless otherwise noted.
2. Sandall English, "Prickly Pear Pleasures," *Arizona Daily Star,* 2 August 1995.
3. Sandall English, "It's Time for Great Prickly Pear Treats," *Arizona Daily Star,* 24 August 1994.
4. Sandall English, *Fruits of the Desert,* (Tucson: Arizona Daily Star, 2000): 30.

Bibliography

The following texts were utilized as points of reference in writing this book.

American Diabetes Association. *101 Tips for Staying Healthy with Diabetes.* Alexandria, Va.: American Diabetes Association, 1996.

American Diabetes Association. *Type 2 Diabetes: Your Healthy Living Guide–Tips, Techniques, and Practical Advice for Living Well with Diabetes.* Alexandria, Va.: American Diabetes Association, 1997.

American Diabetes Association. *The Uncomplicated Guide to Diabetes Complications – What Every Person with Diabetes Should Know about Prevention, Treatment, and Self-care for Complications of the Heart, Nerves, Feet, Eyes, Skin, Kidneys.* Alexandria, Va.: American Diabetes Association, 1998.

Angier, Bradford. *Field Guide to Edible Wild Plants.* Harrisburg, Pa.: Stackpole Books, 1974.

Baker, R. A. "Potential Dietary Benefits of Citrus Pectin and Fiber." *Food Technology* 48 (1994).

Barrett, Amy. "The Cholesterol Sweepstakes." *Business Week,* 28 October 2002.

Beaser, M. D., S. Richard, V. C. Joan, and R. D. Hill. *A Program for Managing Your Treatment: The Joslin Guide to Diabetes.* New York: Fireside, 1995.

Biermann, June, and Barbara Toohey. *The Diabetic's Book: All Your Questions Answered.* New York: G. P. Putnam's Sons, 1994.

Britton, N. L., and J. N. Rose. *The Cactacea: Descriptions and Illustrations of Plants of the Cactus Family.* New York: Dover, 1963.

Chen, M. S., et al. "Prevlence and Risk Factors of Diabetic Retinopathy among Non-Insulin Dependent Diabetes Meillitus," *Opthamolgy* 100 no. 8 (Aug 1993).

Curtin, L. S. M. *By the Prophet of the Earth.* Tucson: University of Arizona Press, 1984.

DiSilvestro, Robert A. "Flavonoids as Antioxidants." In: Wolinsky, Ira, and James F. Hickson, ed. *Handbook of Nutraceuticals and Functional Foods.* Boca Raton, Fla.: CRC Press, LLC, 2001.

Duke, James A., and Alan A. Atchley. *Handbook of Proximate Analysis: Tables of Higher Plants.* Boca Raton, Fla.: CRC Press, 1986.

Ebeling, Walter. *Handbook of Indian Foods and Fibers of Arid America.* Los Angeles: University of California Press, 1986.

Felker, P., and C. E. Russel. "Effects of Herbicides and Cultivation on the Growth of *Opuntia* in Plantations." *Journal of Horticultural Science* 63 no. 1 (1988).

Ford, Karen Cowan. "Las Yerbas De La Gente: A Study of Hispano-American Medicinal Plants." Ann Arbor: University of Michigan Anthropological Papers, 1975.

Forsham, P. H., "Treatment of Type I and Type II Diabetes," *Townsend Letter for Doctors* 53 (Dec 1987): 390–393.

Gruberg, E. R., and S. A. Raymond. *Beyond Cholesterol: Vitamin B6, Arteriosclerosis, and Your Heart.* New York: St. Martin's Press, 1981.

Harrington, H. D. *Edible Native Plants of the Rocky Mountains.* Albuquerque: University of New Mexico Press, 1967.

Hodgson, W. *Edible Native and Naturalized Plants of the Sonoran Desert North of Mexico.* Tempe: Arizona State University, 1985.

King, H., and M. Rewers. "Diabetes in Adults is Now a Third World Problem." *Bulletin of the World Health Organization* 69 no. 6 (1991).

Mayes, Vernon O., and Barbara Bayless Lacy. *Nanise' A Navajo Herbal: One Hundred Plants from the Navajo Reservation.* Tsaile, Ariz.: Navajo Community College Press, 1989.

Millspaugh, Charles F. *American Medicinal Plants: An Illustrated and Descriptive Guide to Plants Indigenous to and Naturalized in the United States Which Are Used in Medicine.* New York: Dover, 1974.

Moyer, Ellen. *Cholesterol & Triglycerides: Questions You Have, Answers You Need.* Allentown, Pa., People's Medical Society, 1995.

Niethammer, Carolyn. *American Indian Food and Lore: 150 Authentic Recipes.* New York: Macmillan Publishing Company, Inc., 1974.

Werbach, M. D., R. Melvyn, and Michael T. Murray, N.D. *Botanical Influences on Illness: A Sourcebook of Clinical Research.* Tarzana, Calif.: Third Line Press, 1994.